What Your Doctor Won't Tell You

What Your Doctor Won't Tell You

The Real Reasons You Don't Feel Good
and What You Can Do About It

DAVID SHERER, M.D.

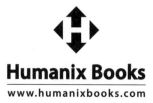

Humanix Books

www.humanixbooks.com

Humanix Books, P.O. Box 20989, West Palm Beach, FL 33416, USA
www.humanixbooks.com | info@humanixbooks.com

Humanix Books is a division of Humanix Publishing, LLC. Its trademark, consisting of the words "Humanix Books," is registered in the Patent and Trademark Office and in other countries.

Disclaimer: The information presented in this book is not specific medical advice for any individual and should not substitute medical advice from a health professional. If you have (or think you may have) a medical problem, speak to your doctor or a health professional immediately about your risk and possible treatments. Do not engage in any care or treatment without consulting a medical professional.

ISBN: 978-1-63006-165-4 (Hardcover)
ISBN: 978-1-63006-164-7 (E-book)

Printed in the United States of America
10 9 8 7 6 5 4 3 2 1

This book is dedicated to all my medical mentors:

William F. McNary, MD
John O'Conner, MD
John McCahan, MD
S. Howard Wittels, MD
Mark Behr, MD
Howard Greenfield, MD
Ronald Kotler, MD
Christopher Tirotta, MD
James J. McDonald, DDS
Samuel Peretsman, MD
Talal Munasifi, MD
Alan Wise, MD
Gordon Avery, MD
John McConnell, MD
Jeff Elliot, MD
Pete Conrad, MD
Arthur Burgerman, MD
John Eng, MD
Stephen Dejter, MD
Neil Stern, MD
Stu Katz, MD
Andrew Astrove, MD
Jean Gilles Tchabo, MD
Emanuel Papper, MD
Robert Gallo, MD
Pam Alexander, MD
and, of course, Max G. Sherer, MD

Contents

Preface

In the late winter of 2017, Executive Vice President and Chief Content Officer of Bottom Line Inc. Marjory Abrams approached me about the prospect of writing a monthly blog on health and medicine for their publication. I had been a friend of the organization for years, offering my expert opinions on a range of related topics, and I was fully in tune to their goal of offering expert-vetted information that would assist their readers. I agreed to the offer and have been writing for them ever since. Marjory and I decided on a concise description of what I had hoped to achieve in my writing and she came up with this:

> Dr. David Sherer is bold enough to tell you what others in the medical profession haven't the courage to say, with inside information on health, healthcare, related public policy and the latest in prevention, diagnosis and treatment of disease.

When she sent me that blurb, I was satisfied about the theme and goals of the blog. Ever since then, I have strived to craft my messages in ways "bold" enough to get people to think carefully about their health habits and to consider changing them for the better. I pride myself in trying to bring new and different approaches to my topics. I hope that after reading this book you will share a similar point of view.

And please note: The material in this book is presented for informational purposes only and should never be used as a substitute for your own personalized medical care. Always consult your personal physician or other healthcare provider when considering any aspect of your medical care, particularly regarding medications, supplements, a change in health habits, and any planned treatments for any ailment. The opinions expressed in this work are just that—opinions—and are not a substitute for personalized medical care.

Introduction

A Perfect Storm

The people of America now stand at a crossroads. Whether they realize it or not, there is a perfect storm brewing that will, within a decade or two, sweep them up in a maelstrom of turbulence related both to their health and their ability to protect that most precious of assets. It is no exaggeration to say that, if the present trends continue, the people of this country will face choices that will either compel them to change their behaviors or doom them to suffer the whims of a broken system.

In my almost 40 years in medicine, I have learned a lot about human biology, human frailty, and human nature. The changes related to so many aspects of health that have emerged in those four decades are discouraging to me as a scientist and a healer, from both a theoretical and practical standpoint. The forces behind those changes are abundantly evident to me as I look back on my vigorous schooling in physiology and pathology. The practical side of the changes are revealed in what I and physicians like me see every day in the clinical setting: a population virtually hell-bent on making themselves sick through the scourge of obesity, the curse of drug and substance abuse, or the nurturing of behaviors that subject us all to a great enemy—excess cortisol.

The great medical writer and physician Siddhartha Mukherjee wrote a best-selling book in which he referred to cancer as "the emperor of all maladies." Along similar lines, I like to refer to obesity as "the mother of all maladies," a condition that, like her offspring hypertension, diabetes, degenerative joint disease, gastrointestinal disease, and a host of others, now riddles our population with infirmity, pain, and untold suffering. It is telling in this regard that in the 1960s in the United States, the average adult male weighed 150 pounds. Today, that number is 200 pounds. Sadly, the consequence of that increase in girth has led to predictable results. A full one-third of American adults are pre-diabetic. The number of prescription drugs the average person in our nation takes keeps growing. It is well-known by medical professionals that although Americans spend more per capita on healthcare than any other nation, their outcomes lag behind many other countries who spend far less. And these statistics appear to worsen with each passing year.

We are an affluent nation, but a sick one. The reasons behind this are complex and daunting. Much of it has to do with a cultural shift in how we see ourselves as living beings trying to function in an ever more stressful and competitive world. But there are other forces at work as well. Madison Avenue and the ad industry have, for the better part of a century, contributed much to the decline in the general health of the nation. This is no mere conspiracy theory babble. The things that companies try to sell us—the fat, sugar, and refined carbohydrate–laden fast-food we eat, the 140 pounds per annum per person of sugar we consume, the foodie culture that places food as circus side-show entertainment (with gut-busting eating contests and the like)—all have a shameful place in the pantheon of health-destroyers. But it goes beyond that. We have, as behavioral science has proven, become literally rewired. Our brains are not the same brains as people who lived even a few decades before us. Our instant world becomes ever more "instant" with the release of the newest smartphone, operating system, or gadget. Our ability to pull ourselves off of machines has become so challenging as to be almost impossible. In prior days, smoking was the habit doctors were trying to get their patients to beat. Now, sadly, it is electronics, and the doctors themselves are as seriously addicted as their patients.

Part of the perfect storm referenced earlier is that Americans are and will likely continue to be a population of aging, chronically ill people. How we as a society are going to deal with that is paramount to our future well-being. Past strides have been made. The first real attempts to marshal government forces to care for the nation's sick, other than local relief agencies, state hospitals, and care for veterans, were the Medicare and Medicaid programs, which began under President Johnson's administration in July of 1965. This more modern-day New Deal, coming decades after President Franklin Roosevelt's programs of reform, recovery, and relief in the aftermath of the Great Depression, was envisioned to assist in providing healthcare for the nation's seniors and indigent. It still does so today, with varying degrees of effectiveness.

But these systems, such as the Veterans Health Administration, the State Children's Health Insurance Program, the Department of Defense TRICARE system, and the Indian Health Service, have received their share of criticism. Paramount among these is perhaps the Veterans Health Administration, where allegations of inefficiency and neglect have plagued that institution for years. And many of the private insurers, the so-called third-party payors that healthcare policy wonks so frequently reference, have earned their share of blame as well. They have been at the center of a political debate, championed by Senator Bernie Sanders of Vermont, who advocates "Medicare for All" and a virtual dismantling of the present healthcare structural architecture.

But whatever else has been done or not done by individual citizens, ad agencies, the federal government, or any number of other players in the present health drama of the nation, one fact is inescapable: We do not merely have a "healthcare crisis" in America. We have a "health crisis," and no amount of spin or rationalization can change that.

If you have deigned to read thus far, you must be curious as to where I am heading. "Is this guy trying to tell me how to live my life?" you might wonder. "Who is he to tell me what to do and not to do when it comes to my health and medical care?" Both are legitimate questions. The answer is: I am not telling you how to live your life or telling you what to do or not do.

What I hope to do in this book, which is based in large part upon my writings and interviews that have appeared in Bottom Line Inc., is to give you enough verifiable information about current medicine, healthcare, and relevant public policy so you can make your own best judgments as to whether a change in your behavior will, if you are inclined, effect a positive change in your life. I want to strip away the veneer of political correctness when it comes to health and give you the basic truths behind the implications of the daily decisions we make that affect our health. These decisions, mostly based on how we approach food, physical activity, our mental and emotional states, our interactions with others, and our approach to accessing healthcare, have profound effects on our physical, mental, and emotional states. Rather than being a book on how to eat, how to exercise, how to shop for a health plan, and so on, this work strives only to inform. Because with information comes power. And with power, there is the potential for positive change.

You can go to untold websites, read myriad books and magazine articles, listen to thousands of podcasts and TED Talks to learn about the latest diet, exercise, emotional, and psychological support strategies, or other "expert" information in an attempt to better your health. My goal here is not merely to add to that body of work.

Rather, I want to tell you what are the often-unmentioned constants behind the causes and effects of our behaviors, actions which, as I have said, translate into the sad overall state of health we see today in our country.

When you go to your doctor's office for a visit, there is a lot that goes unuttered. As the clinician clacks away at the keyboard, you get your 12 minutes to reveal what your problem is, review the medications you are on, undergo a cursory physical exam, and then receive a treatment plan, which may or may not involve blood tests, imaging studies (X-rays, CT scans, and the like), referrals to specialists, or other interventions to deal with your presenting problems. You may get a short lecture to "lose some weight, exercise more, and meditate" if your clinician is really in tune with your problems, and you might even receive a handout encouraging you to do what the doctor says and the best ways to do them.

But in reality, there's no time for you, or the doctor for that matter, to really get behind the issues that probably brought you there: Why are you 40 pounds overweight, why is your cholesterol in a dangerously high range, why do your knees always hurt from the degenerative joint disease exacerbated by your high body mass index?

No, the doctor has to move on to the next patient on her "panel," and you have to rush to the pharmacy to pick up your meds before fighting traffic to get back to your stressful job. There is no time for reflection here—no time to digest the why and how of your visit, of the reasons you got in such a medical mess to begin with. The radio in your car is telling you about this or that $2 triple cheeseburger special offer, your workplace is having a lunch party for a retired colleague catered by the local BBQ joint (with sugary sodas to drink and a preservative-filled sheet cake for dessert from the local grocery store), you have to get those reports finished before you pick up your kid at 5 pm from sports practice, and there's no time to think about how in the world you are going to change the life you are in. You are just too tired and too beaten down to have the energy and will to find out. And so it continues.

My hope is that this book will reveal to you and convince you that small changes can have deep and lasting benefits when it comes to your health. I hope that, once armed with the knowledge in this book, you will be motivated to make the choices necessary to live the healthiest life possible. It is not easy and it is not quick, but it is doable. It will take motivation, willpower, and an ability to think critically and independently, but are you not worth it?

The chapters in this book deal with the major areas of health and medicine that affect physical and mental well-being the most, and which most patients can readily relate to: weight and fitness, medications (including supplements), interaction with your doctor and other medical staff, pain control, how doctors get trained, the root causes of medical errors, the secret language of medicine, a review of our nation's biggest killers, a primer on medical literacy, public policy, and the best and worst trends in health and medicine of the past 50 years. These are admittedly arbitrary and even, some might say, scattered areas to cover. To that I say this: These are the most frequently expressed areas of concern that I have heard in the hundreds of thousands of patient interactions I have had since entering clinical medicine in Boston in 1982. The list is not meant to be comprehensive—that would take volumes and years of research. Rather, these are the topics that I feel are the most important to discuss frankly with you, areas you should carefully and critically examine if you want to improve your health and better deal with a flawed system.

There will be many statistics quoted, many of which are mere estimates. Because there is so much conflicting data out there, I have tried to get my numbers from reliable medical sources, such as respected and mainstream medical websites, renowned medical journals, recognized medical university sources, and the like. You might find that your own research will reveal different but, I suspect, similar statistics. Bear in mind that no one can give exact figures for the topics I cover, only the best educated guesses available.

You might find that my message is blunt and even at times harsh. It is not meant to be the latter. Some people might say, especially with regard to my attitudes about obesity, that I am engaging in "shaming." If that is your take on an honest attempt to offer evidence-based information grounded in solid medical research with the hope of improving your health, then you will find no apology offered by me. It is long past the time, I contend, that political correctness over this serious medical issue, one that insidiously saps the health and financial resources of this nation, be thrown by the wayside and replaced by an unvarnished discussion of the problem.

Once you have read and understood my message, it will be up to you to decide if what I have had to say makes medical sense and if acting upon the information presented would potentially benefit you. I encourage you to talk to your family, your friends, and any medical professionals you might go to or know to get ideas and criticism from them regarding what you've read here. Maybe those people have learned similar things in the mainstream media, books, or from other sources. Perhaps they have differing opinions as to what the best approaches are to improve health. That is all good. It is great to hear all sides of an issue before deciding what might be the right path for you.

But whatever you do, the most important primary message I have for you is this: Think for yourself. For too long, the average person, bombarded by Madison Avenue and the societal norms of diet, physical activity, and other behaviors, has been subliminally guided to self-destructive habits that have cost our American society trillions of dollars and a lot of headache and heartache. I implore you to try your best to resist and thus change for the better. Be aware of what and how you eat, when and to what extent you move and use your body, and how you think. Carefully examine the choices you make every day and see if the evidence I provide rings true in your own life. But most of all, try your best. You will be surprised at what you can do if you think for yourself, make the effort, and tell the health-wrecking powers that be (who often line their pockets at your expense) to get lost.

You will be the better for it.

What Your Doctor Won't Tell You

CHAPTER 1

The 800-Pound American in the Room

The Obesity Threat

I t's no exaggeration: Americans who are overweight or obese put their health at grave risk. *Overweight*, meaning a body mass index (kilograms of weight divided by height in square meters) of 25 to 30, and *obese*, a body mass index of 30 and above, puts you at risk for a host of things you really don't want, including high blood pressure, obstructive sleep apnea, type 2 diabetes, arthritis, asthma, stroke, heart attack, gastro-esophageal reflux, certain types of cancer—the list goes on.

Just as scary as this is the fact that the incidence of overweight/obese people in our country has doubled since 1970. The causes are not hard to figure out: Cheaper "bad for you calories" (fast food, highly processed foods full of lots of sugar, refined carbohydrates, and saturated fats) combined with a more sedentary populace is the perfect recipe for this disturbing trend. A casual perusal on any given busy street, mall, or public venue proves the point: a startling 70% of Americans are either overweight or obese, and the numbers are climbing. A telling fact is that, in the mid-1960s, an average American male weighed about 150 pounds. Today, that number is 200 pounds. This excess body mass, almost always the result of excess fat in relation to muscle and other tissues in the body, has led to epidemic proportions of the diseases and conditions listed earlier. This disturbing trend adds billions of dollars in cost to our healthcare expenditures each year and overwhelms the same delivery system we increasingly depend upon. The peripheral costs are staggering as well. Absenteeism from work, disability costs, increased insurance premiums, and premature death all add up to billions more wasted and spent.

Part of the problem is what I call the "normalization of obesity." The portrayal of the average American in film, commercials, print, and general media as overweight to obese has become more common as the average weight of the populace has gotten larger. Food ads celebrating the relative cheapness of an enormous amount of unhealthy calories, particularly marketed to young-to-middle-aged men, has done much to fuel this problem. The depiction of food itself as a kind of object of lust, desire, and commerciality, rather than nutrition and sustenance (e.g., eating contests, celebrity chef shows, and the like), has contributed to what is a near "pornification" of what used to be merely something to eat or a source of vital nutrition. As well, the attitude that you could always take pills to treat the myriad problems that being overweight/obese present (e.g., the TV ad for the "purple pill" GERD medicine, portraying the obese construction worker who eats as many chili dogs as he likes because he can take an antacid) is all too common in American life.

Until we attack the overweight/obesity problem at its root cause, as former First Lady Michelle Obama tried to do with her children's initiative on the subject, we will not make a dent in the problem. And as we have seen, a serious health and economic problem it is. We, as a society, need to take this problem very seriously, for as this issue gets out of control in our country, as it is in many emerging economies of the world, the morbidity, mortality, and sheer dollar costs will exact a heavy toll.

But despite the overwhelming evidence that being overweight and obese subjects you to the diseases and associated risks I've mentioned, the problem, like the American waistline, only seems to increase with each passing year. Unlike the smoking rate, which has plummeted dramatically since reaching its peak in the 1950s and 1960s, the 25+ BMI subpopulation is stubbornly ensconced in the American populace. Despite the fad diets, exercise routines, supplements, weight-loss regimens, and fitness equipment that get bought, used, and soon discarded, the problem remains like an unwanted house guest. It is truly a national malady.

How Did We Get to This Point?

Where did this problem come from? How is it that the average male in this country is now 33% heavier than his father was in 1965? What does this all mean for our health and economy when one-third of all adults in America are prediabetic?

The answers are many and complex. First and foremost, there's neurobiology. In an enlightening article in *Forbes* magazine in 2013 by Melanie Haiken entitled "The New Theory on Weight Loss: Your Bad Diet Has Damaged Your Brain," the author drew some startling conclusions. In discussions with obesity expert Dr. Louis Arrone, she learned it was the American diet itself that caused changes in the brain, particularly the hypothalamus. She quotes Dr. Arrone as saying that "eating fattening foods causes inflammatory cells to go into the hypothalamus" and that this "overloads the neurons and causes neurological damage." The article goes on to describe research from the University of Liverpool that found that a "diet high in saturated fat and simple carbohydrates sets in motion a chain reaction of 'metabolic dysfunction' involving appetite regulating hormones leptin and ghrelin." Also, the research found that the brain actually undergoes physical changes and that all these factors result in "your brain gone haywire and you can no longer trust the messages it's sending you about hunger, appetite and fullness." In this regard, Dr. Arrone said "It's like your gas gauge points to empty all the time, whether or not the tank is full."

This research and the conclusions drawn from it were game changers, for it elucidated finally that the typical Western diet of refined carbohydrates and heavily saturated fats actually rewired your brain into a dangerous and damaging mode of functioning. Not only are the very things you are eating destructive, but those same fats and carbs were actually programming you to eat more of them. The sword cutting you to metabolic ribbons has, evidently, two very sharp sides to it.

In a nation where the national meal combination has traditionally been a burger with fries and a soda, it's no wonder we are losing the battle against the almighty pound.

Second, there's the sedentary aspect. Kudos to *Forbes* again on this. A 2019 article by Nicole Fisher entitled "Americans Sit More Than Any Time in History and It's Killing Us" referenced work from the Mayo Clinic that reviewed 13 studies, concluding that "those who sat for more than 8 hours a day with no physical activity had a risk of dying similar to the risks of dying posed by obesity and smoking." According to the article, sedentary jobs are up over 80% since 1950, and that research indicates that "too much sitting offset any benefits of working out." The article even covered in detail the problems associated with sitting for long hours at a time in the brain, neck, shoulders, back, abdomen, hips, gluteal muscles, legs, and even the bones.

So a higher than normal BMI and a sedentary lifestyle (which itself contributes to further overweight and obesity problems) are clearly two major players wreaking havoc with your health. So what other weight-related factors are making us sicker?

I've already discussed the dietary brain changes and the fact that we are too immobile for too much of the time. But there are the social factors as well, some subtle and some not. What are they? First there's time, which as we know, waits for no one. Time. The all-elusive entity that we wish we had more of. Since we are all so busy pursuing the American Dream—that is, a consumer-driven ideal that was somehow put on a pedestal and never got taken down—we have suffered for it. We have suffered because the realization of that dream takes money. The best description of consumerism I've ever heard goes something like this: Consumerism is the spending of money we don't have to buy things we don't need to impress people we don't like.

Isn't that the truth? Consumerism and money.

We are all so busy chasing this dream that there's little time for self-care. The same society that fails to see the irony in people literally being crushed to death on Black Friday after Thanksgiving so that some buyer scores a deal on a 76-inch TV (so you can be even more sedentary) is the very same society willing to sacrifice health for "things." Let's face it, climbing the corporate ladder is not now and never has been conducive to salubrious living. Endless meetings, early days, late nights, hours in traffic, taking care of the kids, and the shopping . . . Where's the time and energy left to eat healthfully and get enough exercise? It's small wonder we have a weight problem in this country.

Then there's the normalization of obesity that I spoke about earlier. So embedded and pervasive has the crappy American diet become, replete with saturated fat, highly refined carbohydrates, heavy salt and white sugar, that the depiction of average Americans in television commercials has reflected this growing change. The husband grilling his burgers in the backyard or the woman shilling for her psoriasis medicine during the commercial break on the nightly news are more likely to be of ample girth, as are the random citizens who might appear in a news report whose footage was shot on a busy U.S. city street or town.

The Complications of Obesity

So what else has resulted from the American diet and a sedentary lifestyle? A rise in colon cancer among young people.

I've read and studied the habits of people on the Greek island of Ikaria, who enjoy unparalleled longevity and vigor with their excellent diet and their physically and emotionally connected way of living. People like them, who live in the so-called blue zones around our world, enjoy similar benefits. Blue zones (coined by Dan Buettner in his book, *The Blue Zones*) are regions in the world where an inordinate number of people live healthy lives to very old age, often beyond 100. Sadly, in our own country meanwhile, researchers have found an alarming rise in colon and rectal cancers in Gen X and millennial-aged people in our country. The reasons for this appear to be many.

First, diets that are high in refined sugars and carbohydrates, low in fiber and high in fat, appear to be behind the increase in these cancers. Second, the resultant obesity from high caloric intake and a sedentary lifestyle was also cited by the researchers as possible reasons for the increase. Third, environmental toxins may also be playing a part.

Colon and rectal cancer in people over 55 years of age appears to be decreasing, however. This is probably due to better awareness and screening for the disease. But in younger people, where screening had traditionally not been as vigorous (except in certain at-risk groups, like people who have a family history of cancer or inflammatory diseases of the GI tract), the rise in cancers has come as a shock to many researchers. These findings, which were recently reported in the journal of the National Cancer Institute, have sounded alarm bells among doctors and other scientists who follow these conditions. It has even prompted some to call for earlier screening in these younger at-risk groups.

Traditionally, patients have been taught to report changes in bowel habits to their doctor. These include blood in the stool, changes in the caliber of the bowel movement (particularly pencil-thin stools), mucus or other discharge, or any darkening or other unusual discoloration in the bowel movement. Testing patients for hidden blood in the stool has been a great help in reducing the progression of cancers in patients who may have early stage tumors. Colonoscopy screening has virtually revolutionized the diagnosis and treatment of colon and rectal cancer. But these new findings are causing much discussion on how to deal with this newly found clinical information.

What has not changed are the recommendations that relate to better health and a reduction of many types of cancer in all age groups: a healthy body weight (usually meaning a body mass index of less than 25), daily aerobic exercise and weight training, a diet high in fiber and low in refined sugar and saturated fat, moderate alcohol consumption, and the avoidance of tobacco use. Because many younger people have poor diets and are addicted (through video games, computer and other screen time, etc.) to being sedentary, it will be an uphill battle to get people under 40 off their butts and onto their bikes, into the pool and onto the running track. Perhaps harder will be getting them off soda, junk food, and other dietary abominations that are anathema to good health.

The incidence of cancer in people who live in the blue zones of the world is predictably low. Now, it seems, more than ever, is the time for younger people to decide to act and reverse what has become a surprising and unwelcome trend in cancer prevalence in our country.

Diet Types

I said in the introduction to this book that I won't tell you what to eat. *You* have to tell you what to eat. My goal is to present evidence-based information in order for you to make an informed decision. And there certainly is a lot of information out there. But do understand that the math of weight loss and control is actually quite simple: calories consumed must be fewer than calories expended. It really is that simple. I sometimes think of it like a bank account. Every time you eat well (I'll get to that in a minute) and exercise, you earn credits in that account to take off pounds. Everything you eat takes away those credits. The idea, obviously, is to be continuously earning enough credits to cause a calorie *deficit*. With this desired shortfall of calories, weight comes off. This is the golden rule of weight loss and applies in every situation, save for patients who suffer thyroid, genetic or other medical conditions subjecting them to weight-loss resistance.

Now, because there are untold dietary plans to lose weight, which ones have been shown to be the most effective? After all, there are plant-only diets, intermittent fasting, ketogenic diets (low carb), the "caveman" diet (paleo), the Mediterranean diet, lower fat diets, and scores of pay-as-you-go online, delivered food and other expensive plans. Each of these have their plusses and minuses, and I would encourage you to explore them. But keep in mind the success of whatever plan you choose must be one you can stick with and one that your spouse, partner, kids, or other vested parties can live with as well. Plus, it must fit your lifestyle if you are unwilling to make radical changes in your work and personal life.

Diets that eliminate animal meat and products altogether appear to be the best for you, assuming you can get vital nutrients, including vitamins and minerals, from alternate sources. Vegan diets that are not carefully constructed might leave you deficient in crucial nutrients like vitamin B12, zinc, iodine, calcium, iron, and certain fatty acids. So if you go that route, you would be best served to do your research and/or consult a nutritionist. This regimen is similar to the diet on which former President Bill Clinton was placed after his encounters with cardiac disease and coronary bypass surgery. The Mediterranean diet, so-called because it is based on food from that region rich in fresh vegetables, fruit, whole grains, fish, and olive oil, probably runs a close second in its health benefits. Ketogenic diets like the "South Beach" diet were popular years ago and certainly have a well-deserved reputation for getting weight off quickly. However, there are dangers inherent to the ketogenic diet, some scientists insist. The Harvard School of Public Health revealed that certain long-term effects of a strict ketogenic diet, which is relatively heavy on fats and restrictive of carbohydrates, include an increased risk of kidney stones, osteoporosis, and increased levels of blood uric acid (related to the development of gout). They also question whether the high fat and moderate protein consumption inherent in the keto-genic diet is safe for people with diseases that interfere with normal fat and protein metabolism, such as liver and kidney disorders.

And then there is the paleo diet. Let's look at that for a moment, for it deserves closer examination.

I am riveted by *Sapiens: A Brief History of Humankind* by Yuval Noah Harari. The book is a discussion and analysis of where we humans came from, where we are now, and where we are going. In many ways, the book is vital to understanding how out of sync we are as a species relative to our diets, lifestyles, and activities. And from a health perspective, the book is an eye-opener!

Although *Homo sapiens* is the last remaining of the six human-like species that emerged through evolution, we have done a great job of mucking up our hopes for survival. There is no doubt we are the most intelligent creatures known to have ever lived on this planet. But we are also the most foolish. Foolish enough, with-out question, to threaten our existence with every sort of weapon capable of destroying the planet, as well as pollutants and practices (mining, drilling, etc.) to endanger it. I am not going to discuss the political ramifications of our tribally destructive mentality—just the health ones.

About eight to ten thousand years ago, our ancestors turned from a hunter-gatherer–based lifestyle to a farming one. On first blush that would seem great. It afforded us dependable and consistent food, as well as enabled us to domesticate many animals, including dogs, goats, chickens, and horses. But this farming and domestication came with a price, a price we still pay in our health today.

You see, our former diet and activities as hunter-gatherers depended upon a staple of fruits, seeds, nuts, and lean protein from animal flesh. That diet was, by and large, a very balanced one. Our physical activities—climbing for fruit, digging for tubers and fungus, and running after game—was of the type that fit our bodies' habitus.

But with the advent of farming, our dietary emphasis turned to grain, particularly wheat and corn. Our activities, once domestic animals were around for our protein sources, took a turn for the worse. Farming required clearing land, sowing grain, creating canals and wells for irrigation, burning scrubland and forests to create fields for planting grain, and transporting large stores of crops to villages and towns. This, unlike running and digging, our bodies were not designed to do. Indeed, Harari notes in his book that men and women from the Age of Agriculture showed more skeletal evidence of bone and joint disease than our older ancestors.

"So what?" you may say. "How does that relate to me in the twenty-first century? I can't live like a person who hunted and gathered over 10,000 years ago." Perhaps not. But I contend you can adopt some of the habits of our ancestors and have the best of all worlds: the health benefits of more exercise and better nutrition, along with the advances of modern medicine. Earlier in the book, I discussed the dangers of diets high in simple carbohydrates (mostly in the form of wheat and corn) and sugar (mostly cane sugar and high fructose corn syrup). We have seen that about 70% of Americans, with their sedentary lifestyles, are overweight or obese, partly because we seldom use our bodies in the "functional" ways our hunter-gatherer ancestors did: lots of walking, running, climbing, and so on. So what does this mean?

To me, the message is simple. From a body habitus and fitness standpoint, *Homo sapiens* was much better off in the pre–Agricultural Revolution days, as the author strongly suggests. We can learn from our relatives who lived more than 10,000 years ago by adopting certain imitative habits:

- Vary your diet with fruits, nuts, vegetables, fungus (mushrooms and truffles), lean sources of protein, and whole grains (in reduced amounts).
- Incorporate functional exercise, like walking, running, and even climbing (yes, that's right, climbing). You don't have to climb a tree; a hill, jungle gym, or climbing wall will do.
- Read Harari's book. Learn how the author calls the Age of Agriculture the biggest fraud of all time (you'll see why when you read it).

Does that mean you have to deprive yourself? Not necessarily. After all, life still has to have some sweetness to it, don't you agree? But the 152(!) pounds of added sugar we eat each year is not what I had in mind. Because of the recognized dangers of a high-sugar diet, food industry manufacturers have come up with the all-too-familiar alternatives, recognized by their color-coded packets: the pink, the blue, the yellow, and now the green. The pinks usually contain saccharin, dextrose, and cream of tartar. The blues contain aspartame, dextrose, and maltodextrin. The yellow's primary sweetening ingredients are dextrose, maltodextrin, and sucralose. The pure forms of the green stuff contain stevia leaf extract and erythritol.

So what does this mean for your health? I have my own opinions. Personally, the only stuff I would consider using to sweeten my coffee, tea, or cereal is the green stuff. Here's why.

In my discussion of glycemic index later in this chapter, you will see that certain foods raise your blood sugar by differing degrees, thereby putting varying stresses on your pancreas and the cells that make insulin. The value 100 is arbitrarily assigned, 2 hours post-ingestion, to glucose as the ingested product. High glycemic index values are considered to be above 70, mid-range is 56 to 69, and low is considered below 55. The following are the indexes for different sweeteners:

- Maltodextrin 110
- Dextrose 100
- Sucralose 0
- Aspartame 0
- Stevia 0
- Saccharin 0
- Erythritol 1
- Agave 17
- Honey 60 to 74, depending upon variety

Leaving all the other arguments aside about the alleged safety or dangers of aspartame, saccharin, and other artificial sweeteners, I would prefer using a sweetener that had a low or nonexistent glycemic index and one that comes naturally, from a plant. The answer here should be clear.

Worthy of mention here is the increasing popularity of monk fruit, whose extract has been used as an effective sweetener for drinks and foods. Its glycemic index is zero, and studies in mice have even revealed the potential for lowering blood sugar and cholesterol levels, as well as the possibility of antioxidant and anti-inflammatory effects.

But leaving sweeteners aside, whatever diet or eating plan you choose, consider these basic principles based on evidence that it's beneficial to greatly or completely eliminate these things forever from your diet: anything white (white rice, potatoes, white bread, and flour), sodas of any kind (including diet), meat that is fatty, fruit juices that are laden with sugar (apple and orange are big culprits), and alcohol in excess of one drink per day. Watch your portion size, because this is a big waistline killer. A meat serving should be about the size of your palm. If you must eat processed foods, try to consume store-bought pre-prepared food with less than five listed ingredients. The more rich, natural color in the food you eat, the more antioxidants it is likely to contain, and antioxidants are great for you. Cherries, eggplants, and kale are good examples. It's really just that simple.

But to repeat, it's up to *you* to decide, probably after some concentrated research and a review of your own health situation, what is best for you. If you can, enlist the help of your doctor or a dietitian or nutritionist, if you have access to ones who will engage actively and carefully. But the important thing is to do it, not merely think of doing it. With an hour a day of exercise, meaning at least 40 minutes of cardio (walking, jogging, swimming, tennis, etc.) and 20 minutes of resistance training and core work (hand weights and abdomen and back work), and a diet plan you can live with, the pounds will come off and you will increase your chances for a better, longer, and fuller life. Do your research and get started. Pick an eating plan and buy some workout shoes, a mat, a jump rope, and some hand weights. That's your gym right there, all for less than a hundred bucks.

Blood Sugar and Diabetes

Each January, people make resolutions that will be broken by Valentine's Day. However, if you plan to keep one resolution right this minute, let it be this: Don't be a mindless stooge or lemming. The unhealthy and high glycemic-index (see further on in this chapter) American diet is terrible for you. Whenever possible, the consumption of unrefined, whole-fiber carbohydrates that still have their husks and grains is much more desirable and healthful. These grains cause the gradual rise in blood sugar and thus prevent the spike in insulin that so depletes our already assaulted pancreases, thus giving that vital organ a much-deserved rest. Your pancreas has only enough insulin-producing cells to last one lifetime.

Relevant to any discussion of insulin and diet are the concepts of *glycemic index* and *glycemic load*, two parameters that have received increased attention over the years. As I mentioned before, the first parameter is described as a value assigned to food between 0 and 100, with 100 representing the relative blood glucose value rise 2 hours after consuming pure glucose. A food is said to have a low GI (glycemic index) at ranges of 55 or less, high if 70 or more, and be mid-range if between 56 and 69. The GL (glycemic load) represents, as expressed by a number, how much the ingested food will increase a person's serum glucose level after it is eaten. A formula that relates the two is: grams of carbohydrate in food × GI ÷ 100 = GL. For a single serving of food, a GL larger than 20 is said to be high, 11 to 19 is medium, and less than 10 is low.

Of note is the fact that studies have linked a lower GI and GL diet to a lesser risk of developing type II diabetes.

But to help save your own life, to mitigate, delay, or avoid altogether the curses of obesity and all the mentioned maladies that go with it, you must actively resist the onslaught of Madison Avenue and the ad industry. Hired by junk-food and fast-food companies, they want nothing more than for you to ingest (and thereby get addicted to) their poison and force you to compensate for your evils with medication, so their sister industry, big pharma, can throw more business their way. Junk and fast-food makers hire advertising companies dying to hook you on health-killers: soda, refined foods, sugar-laden snacks, fat-laden fast food, you name it. Then to clean up the mess created by eating this garbage, the drug companies want to sell you their side-effect-inducing treatments. (Notice I did not say "cure," because that only you can do.) What a mess. It's as true today as it was when I was a kid in the 1960s.

To reiterate, with over 70% of us overweight, and one in three adults being prediabetic in America, it is now virtually assumed that poor lifestyle habits are just part and parcel of daily living, along with the attitude that medicines are the natural and expected solutions to our gluttony and sloth. This attitude is dangerous but resistible. It's not too late. I write and speak on this over and over again. Eat better. Move your body. Control your stress. These are the three pillars of better health. Focus more on that than "achievement."

What good is a high-powered job if you are sick?

What use are material things if you are not around to use them?

Is the cost to your health, your relationships, and your well-being worth the things we chase and sacrifice in order to be, in society's eyes, a success?

Don't be Madison Avenue's stooge or big pharma's lemming. Think for yourself. Make the commitment to consider it unacceptable and undesirable to do as others do: to overeat, to be lazy, and to be careless with your most precious commodity. Follow my advice and save your own life.

CHAPTER 2

Medication Nation

A Flawed Solution

Harry Moseley Stevens, an Englishman whose life spanned half of the ninteenth century and a third of the twentieth century, was a sporting event concessionaire who sold scorecards to attendees of sporting events. (He was also the alleged inventor of the hot dog, but that's another story.) He coined the famous phrase: "You can't tell the players without a scorecard!" The scorecards, and the hot dogs, made him a wealthy man.

Unlike in Harry Stevens's day, currently your doctor can likely tell his patients from a scorecard of their medications. A study reported a few years back by researchers at Mayo Clinic and Olmsted Medical Center revealed that 70% of Americans take at least one prescription medicine, and many take more than one, with an impressive 20% taking five or more. When you add up all the vitamins and supplements people are taking, you'd be hard-pressed to find any adult American who isn't being medicated with something. What's so telling about this disturbing trend is that oftentimes doctors don't even need to examine you or ask you questions. They can merely look at your medical record and see what medications you are on

17

to understand (most) of your problems and issues. And as I keep saying, most of these problems and issues are, like the proverbial accidental gunshot wound, self-inflicted.

In her illuminating and cogent 2004 book *The Truth About the Drug Companies: How They Deceive Us and What to Do About It*, Marcia Angell, the former editor in chief of the prestigious *New England Journal of Medicine* (and alumnus of my own medical school) had this to say:

> In my view, we have become an overmedicated society. Doctors have been taught only too well by the pharmaceutical industry . . . to reach for the prescription pad. Add to that the fact that most doctors are under great time pressure because of the demands of managed care, and they reach for that pad very quickly. Patients have been well taught by the pharmaceutical industry's advertising. . . . If they don't leave the doctor's office with a prescription, the doctor is not doing a good job. The result is that too many people end up taking drugs when there may be better ways to deal with their problems.

I can think of no better synopsis of the prevailing attitudes that patients hold regarding the role of the doctor and the hoped-for outcome of a typical medical visit.

I've discussed the reasons why Americans have to take so many medications: our terrible diets; sedentary lifestyles and substance abuse; the constant social, financial, and other stresses of modern life—all of which have exacerbated whatever genetic and other predispositions people have for developing a specific illness.

While we attack our bodies with cortisol (built up from chronic stress) and ruin our vascular, musculoskeletal, gastrointestinal, and endocrine systems with inactivity and bad diets, it is small wonder that the majority of prescriptions people take are related to those conditions. Indeed, the top medicines taken in the twenty-first century for people's ills relate to:

- High blood pressure
- Diabetes
- Anxiety, depression, and other mental illnesses
- Stomach and other GI ailments
- Arthritis and other musculoskeletal problems
- Coronary artery disease and high blood cholesterol and lipids
- Management of stroke prevention with blood thinners
- Neurologic diseases such as multiple sclerosis and Parkinson's
- Bacterial and viral infections
- Asthma, chronic obstructive pulmonary disease, and other lung diseases
- Autoimmune disorders
- Chronic pain

That's only a partial list of conditions that often require medical therapy. The costs of these diseases and drugs are staggering, as is the fact that patients often misuse their medications. Nearly $2.7 trillion was spent on healthcare in 2012, but $213 billion could have been saved by diagnosing diseases earlier and using prescription medicine in better ways, according to a report from the IMS Institute for Heath and Informatics. IMS arrived at the $213 billion figure based on six categories in which doctors, patients, or both could be making better use of medication, from getting a prompt diagnosis when new symptoms arise to taking medicines as directed by the doctor. Across the six categories, the researchers generally focused on spending on a handful of common or very expensive diseases—from high cholesterol and blood pressure to HIV and diabetes—for which costs of care and complications are well-documented.

"There's even larger avoidable costs if we were to look at all disease areas" where patients aren't getting optimal care, Murray Aitken, the institute's executive director, told the Associated Press in an exclusive interview. "There's a big opportunity for improvement." Aitken also said more appropriate use of medication—taking each exactly as prescribed, not taking antibiotics for viral illnesses, preventing medication errors and the like—could prevent six million hospitalizations, four million trips to the emergency room, and 78 million visits to doctors and other outpatient care providers each year.

The report, titled "Avoidable Costs in Healthcare," found that the biggest area of waste is patients not taking medicines prescribed by their doctor, either at all or as directed. IMS estimates the cost of such "nonadherence" at about $105 billion a year. Reasons for the longstanding problem include patients fearing drug side effects, not understanding complications that can occur without treatment, having mental health issues, and not being able to afford their medicines.

So whether you are taking statins for cholesterol and lipids, beta blockers, calcium channel blockers, ACE inhibitors, ARBs for high blood pressure, PPIs or antacids for your GERD and stomach, SSRIs or SNRIs for depression and anxiety, or acetaminophen, NSAIDS, or steroids for your joint pains, it's good for both you and your doctor to "tell the players" in your medication lineup, review them during each visit, go over any side effects or interactions you need to look out for, and most important, figure out health behaviors to enable you to get off of as many medications as possible.

The Prices We Pay

However, getting back to the root causes of why we take so many medicines is really the focus of this chapter, as is the perils of taking so many drugs. We've discussed the basic and essential reasons in Chapter 1 for America's (and most of the developed world's) dependency on prescription medication. But to fully understand the full impact of the problem, we must also turn our attention to the price we pay for being hooked on these drugs.

The Western medical model that prevails in the United States, Europe, the United Kingdom, and much of the rest of the developed world is based on allopathic medicine, which refers to that discipline of medical science and practice that is based on research, honed by evidence, and that employs pharmaceuticals and surgical intervention to treat, mitigate, or cure disease. The vast majority of medical schools in those countries train their graduates to adhere to and ensure continuance of that model of care. Sure, there are alternative therapies that many of these doctors have come to embrace, such as acupuncture and traditional Asian or Chinese medicine, homeopathy, herbal medicine, osteopathic manipulation and so on, but by and large the primary allopathic construct still prevails. The whole system of care is based on the assumption that because so many humans, when presenting with a host of lifestyle factors related to diet, activity, and mental and psychological stressors, develop the common "Western diseases" that plague us, research and therefore treatment have been tailored to ameliorate those conditions.

A perfect example is type 2 or "adult onset" diabetes. Hundreds of years ago, this disease was virtually a nonentity (not necessarily so for type 1 or "juvenile onset" diabetes), because people had neither the money nor the opportunity to overeat the kind of food I maligned earlier, nor the type of job or daily lifestyle that would have permitted such a sedentary existence. Certainly, there were obese people back then, but that was the exception rather than the norm that it is today. Perhaps the most famous exception one can find is that of King Henry the Eighth of England, who was a strapping, athletic youth in his early years, only to become the obese, disabled diabetic who was constantly plagued by a chronically infected leg ulcer.

Another example is that of lung cancer, a relatively rare clinical condition centuries ago, but one that exploded in the West once widespread tobacco abuse became rampant. And while it is true that people lived shorter lives in those times and therefore never reached the age to develop many of the diseases we suffer, research has shown that even age-adjusted prevalence of the diseases I've mentioned occur more frequently as our health habits deteriorate.

And what of the apparent explosion of autoimmune diseases that seem to increase in prevalence with each passing year? There is evidence that the presence of manmade chemicals, relatively new to the human organism, and present in our food, water, air, and soil, have caused our bodies to reject them as foreign invaders. As our immune systems attack these alien molecules, our tissues literally become "innocent bystanders" and get caught in the crossfire, resulting in the often debilitating rheumatologic (joint and connective tissue), neurologic (think multiple sclerosis, Parkinson's disease, and ALS), and other autoimmune diseases we see.

Meds and More Meds

So what are we to make of all this? It will be useful to examine the major classes of drugs involved. Then by looking at what they do for us and against us, we can formulate an argument as to why getting off of them is so important. This is so important that I have no doubt most of you take at least one, and probably two or more, of these types of drugs.

GoodRx, a prescription medication web and app service, recently featured the ten most prescribed medications in their annual report of the first quarter of 2019. They were:

1. Atorvastatin (Lipitor)
2. Levothyroxine (Synthroid)
3. Lisinopril (Prinivil, Zestril)

4. Gabapentin (Neurontin)
5. Amlodipine (Norvasc)
6. Hydrocodone/acetaminophen (Vicodin, Norco)
7. Amoxicillin (Amoxil)
8. Omeprazole (Prilosec)
9. Metformin (Glucophage)
10. Losartan (Cozaar)

One of these medications is used to treat high blood lipids (cholesterol and triglycerides), three are for hypertension (high blood pressure), one is for neuropathic pain, one for acute pain, one for GERD and ulcer disease, one for low thyroid, one to kill bacteria (an antibiotic), and one for type 2 diabetes. As you can see, in the case of the blood lipid medication, much of that is to treat deficiencies in diet and lifestyle, although there can be hereditary causes for uncontrollably high blood fats (lipids). Ditto the blood pressure medicines, as obesity, stress, and a lack of fitness are big contributors to that condition as well. In the case of the stomach medication, stress and obesity are big contributors, as is a bacterial infection from the organism *Helicobacter pylori*, which has been recognized in the development of stomach ulcers. The neuropathic pain medicine is often used to treat diabetic pain and pain from autoimmune diseases, both linked to poor health habits and possible exposure to chemical toxins. The acute pain medicine listed has a wide application in pain relief, and the low thyroid medicine can be used for treating low thyroid states due to a genetic predisposition or an autoimmune thyroid disease.

But the list of most prescribed medications proves my point: Many are targeted to treat conditions that affect the vascular system, the heart and all the blood vessels that deliver oxygen-rich blood to all the tissues of your body. The statin in the number one drug spot on the list, and the blood pressure medications in the three, five, and ten spots, are revealing in that these medications are often used to clean up the mess left after a bad diet and health habits have prevailed for too long. Further proof is offered by a recent Centers for Disease Control (CDC) list of the top killers in the United States that places heart disease at number 1 with 647,457 annual deaths, followed by cancer at number 2 with 599,108 deaths.

Target Organs

Before I discuss the merits of lowering blood lipids and the role of inflammation, it's crucial to understand the target organ most affected by the nation's top life-taker, and it's probably not what you think. The next time you are at a cocktail party and feeling full or yourself, ask a group of people what the largest organ in the body is. If they have pondered this before, most people will say the liver or, if they think they are really clever, the skin. These are typical answers, along with the brain, the spleen, and even the intestines. But the answer will surprise you.

The largest organ in the body is the vascular endothelium (i.e., the lining of your blood vessels). This is the inner layer of all your arteries, veins, and capillaries. Indeed, so large is this layer of organ tissue that, if laid flat, it would cover six and a half tennis courts! Astonishing!

Why is this important? Well, that's simple. Cardiovascular disease continues to kill and disable more people in the Western world (and others) than any other disease. It is the leading cause of death and disability due to stroke, heart attack, peripheral vascular disease, and related diseases and conditions such as diabetes, obesity, and high blood cholesterol and other lipids. Billions of dollars are spent each year in the Western world to treat these conditions.

The vascular endothelium is not just an inert barrier layer of cells—they serve many important functions, like releasing important chemicals related to the endocrine (glandular) system, blood clots, inflammation, antioxidants, and other vital functions. This crucial plumbing layer is perhaps the most battered organ in our bodies, abused by our busy lifestyles, poor diets, lack of exercise, stress, smoking, substance abuse, and other factors.

The essential mechanism by which this vital layer is damaged is rather simple: Our genetics and/or our lifestyle choices create a toxic and turbulent environment for this delicate layer of cells, creating micro-tears and inflammatory damage that attracts platelets—the blood elements that not only protect us from uncontrolled bleeding but when sticking to the damaged inner layer of blood vessels cause blockages due to the buildup of cholesterol and other lipid plaques. These plaques block blood flow and lead to poor oxygen delivery to our other organs and tissues. Doctors write millions of prescriptions each year for lipid-lowering medications, heart- and blood pressure–related medicines, anti-inflammatories, diabetes medicines, and others that help mitigate this assault on our plumbing layer. There seems no end in sight to this onslaught.

The answers integral to stopping this attack on our largest organ are ones I've already covered: diet, exercise, and a true cultural shift in the attitude of what is and isn't acceptable for the maintenance of one's health. In theory, the answers are simple, but the application of the answer is difficult. My mantra remains the same: Reduce inflammatory foods (refined, high in sugar and saturated fat), reduce stress (meditation, mindfulness, yoga, strong interpersonal relationships), stop smoking and substance abuse, get one hour of exercise a day that includes both aerobic and resistance training to maintain a healthy body weight, drink alcohol in moderation, and if all else fails, use supplements and prescription medicines. We know all too well the prescription medicines I'm referring to on this list that treat the result, not the cause, of the problem, when disease is due to poor lifestyle choices and not unfortunate genetics alone: cholesterol-lowering, anti-hypertensive, diabetic medicines, and so on.

The supplements that are of potential benefit, with your doctor's approval, include aspirin, fish oil, garlic, coenzyme Q, turmeric, apple cider vinegar, chromium picolinate, biotin, cinnamon, magnesium, hawthorn extract, and others. These supplements, when used alone or together, have varying anti-inflammatory, blood sugar– and blood pressure–lowering, blood thinning and metabolic properties that assist in combatting the vascular-damaging effects of our lifestyles. Do your research, talk with your doctor and nutritionist, if you have access to one, and formulate a plan.

But as with any plan to improve health, this requires commitment. Just understanding the issues is half the battle. Again, it is up to each of us to treat the root cause and not merely the end result of our bodily abuse to effect real change. It is doable, but it involves sacrifice and is difficult. As I've repeated many times in my writings and lectures, I have no delusions that to many this advice will fall on deaf ears. But if just a few people adopt this approach, it will have been worth it.

Bad Cholesterol and Other Problems

Although there is a strong focus on getting cholesterol levels down, more broadly oriented research has shown that cholesterol may not be the only culprit in the development of cardiovascular disease. Practically everyone concerned with heart health has heard that high cholesterol levels in your blood can be a cause of heart and blood vessel disease. But did you know that researchers and doctors are just as concerned with inflammation as a cause of cardiovascular disease? You might ask, "What does inflammation have to do with heart attacks and strokes?" The answer might surprise you.

A few decades ago, researchers studied inflammatory markers, particularly C-reactive protein (CRP), and found that the presence of high levels of these chemicals in the blood can be a good predictor of the development of coronary artery disease, heart attacks, and strokes. Doctors had long known of the correlation of high subtypes of cholesterol in the blood (particularly LDL, or "bad cholesterol") with those conditions, but a series of studies elucidated in the *New England Journal of Medicine* brought out the importance of CRP and the role of inflammation in cardiovascular disease.

It turned out that risk factors associated with cardiovascular disease and high "bad" cholesterol were the same for the high levels of CRP—that is, obesity, high blood pressure, smoking, diabetes, a diet lacking complex carbohydrates that is high in saturated fat and refined sugars, lack of exercise, excessive alcohol use, and genetic factors.

All the factors except genetic ones are under our control, so through lifestyle modification and, when needed, drug therapy, the rates of most cardiovascular disease can be reduced with careful and thoughtful medical care and self-care. However, with the revelation that inflammation and its subsequent damage to the layer of cells lining all our blood vessels can cause heart attacks, strokes, and heart disease, we have new and better ways to fight this major killer.

When the cellular linings of our blood vessels (the endothelium) get inflamed, the surface gets roughed up to the point that a chemical reaction takes place. Through a cascade of chemical and physical events that scientists now better understand, a blockage (known as plaque) builds up and restricts blood flow and thus delivery of vital oxygen to the tissues of the heart, brain, and body. This, in turn, can lead to heart attack, stroke, and other vascular-related diseases. By taking steps to reduce inflammation, we can mitigate many, if not all, of this reaction and lead healthier lives. These steps, which used to focus primarily on reducing LDL cholesterol, now apply to CRP as well, and there are even steps specifically aimed at reducing CRP that we can take. The steps to reduce LDL and CRP are:

• Cessation in the use of all tobacco products

- Improving your diet—with low refined sugar, complex carbs, and foods rich in omega 3s (fish, nuts, avocado, using olive oil instead of butter)
- Exercising
- Getting your blood sugar and blood pressure under control
- Meditation, doing tai-chi or other mind-relaxing techniques
- Controlling stress
- Considering medication as a last resort when all else fails

Steps particularly good for CRP reduction include the previous list, plus:

- Adding turmeric, ginger, flaxseed, and krill oil as supplements
- Indulging in dark chocolate as a midday treat
- Talking to your doctor about measuring your CRP. Less than 1 milligram/liter is good, 1–3 is higher risk, and greater than 3 is a cause for concern.
- Discussing the role of anti-inflammatory medicine, such as aspirin, with your doctor
- Avoiding ultra-carbohydrate-restricting diets such as the once-popular Atkins diet. Such regimens have actually been found to increase CRP in many patients. Choose complex carbs such as whole grains, fruits, vegetables, and high-fiber-content foods that actually lower CRP.

It used to be that cholesterol got all the attention in the cardiovascular medicine arena. But doctors now know, from extensive research over the past two decades, that inflammation and CRP may play as big a role in the development of heart disease and stroke.

And where does diabetes stand in all this? Many of you probably think that diabetes or "high blood sugar" is primarily a metabolic or endocrine (glandular) disorder, and you'd be right. But what many people fail to realize is that diabetes is very much a vascular disease, for it is the high levels of blood glucose, as well as other subtle changes in vascular biology, that create the damage to the "target" organs—the eyes, kidneys, blood vessels, nervous system, and other vital organ systems and that lead to often profound illness and disability. So it is not surprising that diabetics are typically on both blood-sugar-, blood-pressure-, and blood-lipid-lowering medications as well. Keep in mind that the diabetic state is a highly inflammatory one for the body and that the body and its tissues are being attacked from all sides in many deleterious ways.

So now that we understand the damage done to organs most assaulted by the Western lifestyle, let's look at the price we pay for being on these medicines. First, there's the financial cost, which all of you who take these drugs know too well. Perhaps more important, there are the potential side effects, unwanted physiologic changes that come as a result of having to take these agents. In the case of statins, people who take them can most likely tell you about them: muscle aching and weakness, trouble sleeping, abdominal pain and bloating and liver pathology, inflammation of muscular tissues, changes in bowel habits, vertigo or a sense of imbalance, and even skin changes. There are even reports of statins contributing to the development of type 2 diabetes, outright liver damage, memory loss and confusion, and potentially dangerous interactions with other medicines. Do you really want to have to deal with these possibilities?

In the case of blood pressure medications, the scope of side effects depends on the class of antihypertensive, the dose, and your own genetics and body chemistry. The most common complaints are sexual dysfunction and impotence, fatigue, cough, swelling of the lips and airway, light-headedness, headache, nausea and vomiting, drowsiness, and a generalized lack of energy. With metformin, the common type 2 diabetes agent, common complaints are nausea, change in bowel habit, vomiting, and flatulence. The most dangerous potential side effect is lactic acidosis, where too much lactic acid builds up in the blood, causing a dangerous drop in the serum and tissue pH level, negatively affecting so many normal physiologic functions.

The other drugs on the list, the acute painkillers, the acid reducer, and the neuropathic pain medication have side effects of their own, none of which you want. The narcotics can cause respiratory depression, itching, urinary retention, constipation, mental confusion, and drowsiness. The gabapentin is known for drowsiness and fatigue, as well as fever, dizziness, and sedation. Omeprazole can cause headache, dizziness, abdominal pain, nausea, and rashes. The potential side effects of the last listed medication, an essential replacement for people with low thyroid hormone levels, relate mostly to a therapeutic overdose: heart rhythm problems, heart attack, nervousness, muscular spasms, irritability, insomnia, weight loss, diarrhea, weakness, and heat intolerance.

In fairness, not all of these effects are frequent and can occur with varying frequency depending on your own metabolism, genetics, and "body chemistry." But they do occur enough of the time to make taking these medications on a long-term basis a daunting challenge for many patients. It's best not to be on any of them altogether.

Certainly, a list of the most prescribed medications to treat blood pressure elevation, diabetes, abnormal blood lipids, autoimmune and other low-thyroid states, esophageal reflux and high stomach acid conditions, and acute and neuropathic pain represent only a portion of the millions and millions of prescriptions written each year in the United States and worldwide. There are, of course, other widely prescribed medications that treat a variety of ailments: insulin for type 1 diabetes, biologics and monoclonal antibodies for certain cancers and autoimmune diseases, antidepressants, antianxiety medications and antipsychotics for psychiatric disorders, corticosteroids, anti-inflammatories, antibiotics, antivirals, medications to treat neurodegenerative diseases like Parkinson's, dementia, and multiple sclerosis—the list goes on. However, by examining the top ten list, we can discover those ailments that most plague our society and thus understand what is behind the major illnesses that cost us all so dearly.

Now that we understand that poor choices in diet and lifestyle, environmental toxins, unchecked mental and emotional stress, and the hyperproduction of cortisol (the primary stress hormone) lurk at the root of many "Western" ailments, we can also appreciate the price we must pay to treat those conditions under the allopathic care model. So much has been written in the past few decades about alternative therapies, and I would encourage you to look into them if you feel you might benefit. But they are not my focus here, as those methods of healing, be they mind–body based (yoga, meditation, etc.), interventional (like acupuncture and massage), herbal, homeopathic, and others, could fill books on their own. My goal is to get you to follow the simple advice I've repeated ad nauseum, advice targeted to get you to shift your attitude and make simple changes that, through hard work and discipline, reap great rewards.

Supplements

Any discussion of getting off prescription medication would not be complete without mentioning supplements of which almost 80% of the American populace take regularly. These include not only vitamins and minerals, but other plant-based agents as well. In 2019, the Council for Responsible Nutrition reported that 77% of Americans take supplements, with the highest consumption (81%) in adults ages 35–54. They go on to say that the most popular category of supplement were vitamins and minerals, followed by specialty supplements, herbals and botanicals, sports nutrition supplements, and finally weight-management supplements.

Because the use of supplements for health could easily fill its own book as well, I would like to mention only a few that have found favor in treating the cardiovascular, inflammatory, and other general health categories that were represented in our top ten list earlier. Be sure to always check with your doctor or other healthcare provider before starting any supplement, and never change any prescription medication regimen without consulting your doctor first. Because the prescription meds have *their* top ten list, I've come up with my own:

1. Fish oil and other beneficial fatty acids
2. Biotin
3. Chromium picolinate
4. Cinnamon
5. Magnesium
6. Red beets
7. Niacin
8. Garlic
9. Apple cider vinegar
10. Turmeric

I will not go into extensive detail on each of these agents, but I have included them here because of their relative safety, the evidence of their benefit, and their reasonable price. Again, always check with your doctor or provider before considering using these supplements.

Fish oil contains omega-3 fatty acids, as well as some amounts of vitamins A and D. Evidence has shown potential heart benefits through improvements in cholesterol profiles, as well as triglycerides. There are purported blood pressure benefits too, as well as some evidence to support an improvement in heart rhythm problems. (There is no compelling evidence that it will prevent strokes or heart attacks.)

Biotin has been purported to foster health in hair and nails, have a beneficial effect on cholesterol, and help regulate blood sugar.

Chromium assists in modulating the effect of insulin, a hormone involved in blood sugar regulation. Some improvement in blood sugar levels have been reported with its use. The same holds true for cinnamon.

Magnesium is a naturally occurring element present in our blood and tissues and is primarily known to modulate nerve and muscle function. There is even a possible antidiabetic effect, and it may help with migraines and anxiety, too.

Red beet consumption has been linked to a lowering of blood pressure and potential improvements in athletic performance.

Both niacin and garlic have been associated with better blood lipid levels, although in the case of niacin, unpleasant and potentially serious side effects, such as hot flashes, flushing of the skin, and even liver toxicity, have been reported.

The last on my all-star list, turmeric, is a spice that has received a lot of attention in recent years for its potential in reducing the impact of autoimmune diseases and for its antioxidant and anti-inflammatory qualities.

Please understand that these are not the only benefits of these "all-star" members; I encourage you to research them further and see if you and your doctor can find potential benefits in their use. Do realize that some of these agents, particularly niacin, can come with significant unwanted effects, so be aware to look out for those when you weigh the pros and cons.

But consider this: With a commitment to think and therefore live differently, you'll have a reasonable chance of getting off some or all of your prescription medications, with or without the help of some supplements. I hope that prospect excites you.

Incidentally, I saw a cartoon on the web that perfectly describes most patients' attitudes about taking prescription medication versus making an effort to change their habits. It pictured two lines and two service windows. The first service window had a sign over it that read "PILLS AND SURGERY." The other window had a sign above that read "LIFESTYLE CHANGE." There were about 50 people in the first line, and no one in the second.

CHAPTER 3

Is the Cure Worse Than the Disease?

The Potential Dangers of Medical Interventions

Not long ago, a widely read and studied report made disturbing claims that the leading cause of death in the United States is the American medical system. Medicare's recent announcement that it will no longer reimburse hospitals for the cost of treating certain "serious preventable events," such as an object left in a patient's body after an operation, giving a patient mismatched blood, and even the development of certain infections, indicates how bad things have gotten in healthcare and how seriously the government views the problem.

Within the report, the authors attributed nearly 800,000 deaths each year to medical interventions, in contrast to approximately 650,000 deaths from heart disease and 550,000 from cancer. The methodology they used to calculate that number didn't stand up to some observers' analyses, so perhaps the numbers are not quite so high. However, it did get my attention because the statistics came from recognized sources, including peer-reviewed medical journals that cited, for instance, 106,000 deaths annually from adverse drug reactions, 98,000 from medical errors, and 88,000 from infections. Compare this with 160,000 deaths from lung cancer each year. Deaths happen, of course, but preventable deaths from hospital-acquired infections, especially if due to poor hygiene, such as those transmitted by not washing hands, are particularly egregious.

My contention is that although this report is controversial and somewhat alarmist, it has elements of truth. Statistics can always be arranged and interpreted in different ways, but the indisputable point here is that medical errors and complications or adverse effects from medical interventions have reached a crisis point in this country—one that needs to be addressed. That's beginning to happen.

Before I go into more detail, you might want to read my 2020 book from Humanix Books, *Hospital Survival Guide: The Patient Handbook to Getting Better and Getting Out*. That work has expanded sections related to some of the material presented in this chapter.

Let's examine what's behind this alarming trend and how we can protect ourselves.

What Is Behind the Rise of Medically Related Deaths?

At first glance, one might think that doctors, nurses, and other medical professionals have suddenly and inexplicably become inattentive, careless, and even reckless. That's far too simple (and unlikely) an explanation. Instead, it's probable that the alarming statistics are due to a number of different factors, such as the following:

- The American public is getting older and sicker. Growing numbers of aging baby boomers are developing the diseases commensurate with their advanced years and lifestyle choices—heart disease, diabetes, orthopedic problems, and so on. In the meantime, in people of all ages, growing rates of obesity contribute to these same health challenges. More sick people mean more medical interventions—and in hard numbers that adds up to more mistakes or complications.

- In the kind of medical "perfect storm" I mentioned in the Introduction of this book, as more Americans are developing serious health problems, we're struggling with a shortage of medical support personnel, including both doctors and nurses, which decreases the attention paid to patient needs and details of treatment. Also, the ever-increasing complexity of managed care has meant doctors have less time to devote to patients during office visits and as a result are less likely to know the particulars of their history. This sets up a system ripe for medical mistakes.

- Americans today take more prescription medications than anyone else in the world—and drug companies are working hard to get us to take even more. Spending on direct-to-consumer drug advertising has increased over 300% in nearly a decade, to $4.2 billion in 2005 from $1.1 billion in 1997. With that much money aimed at advertising drugs not just to save lives, but to enhance moods or correct erectile dysfunction or alleviate restless leg syndrome, drugs are often being taken by people who don't need them to extend their lives. More drugs mean more adverse reactions and interactions to juggle than ever before—again, creating many more opportunities for errors.

- Although we're paying closer attention to medical errors and preventable complications—paradoxically, the harder we look for them, the more we find. This makes the numbers look worse in the short run, but in the long run this increased vigilance and accountability should result, in theory, in better outcomes.

How Can You Protect Yourself?

There are many preventive actions you can take to shield yourself and your loved ones from this epidemic of deaths related to medical interventions. The doctor's office is a great place to start, because for many people this is their first entry into the medical system. But even then, there are challenges. We have all heard this before. "I went to see the doctor and it was like I was talking to a wall." Or "My doctor seems like he can't wait to get me out of the exam room and move on to the next patient."

Indeed, patients today are frustrated and even angry about their perceived or real miscommunication with their doctors. In many cases, this is justified. Studies have shown that, on average, it takes only 12 seconds for your doctor to interrupt you as you are describing what brought you to his/her attention. But it doesn't have to be this way.

Encounters with doctors are now at an all-time high. This means the system that is supposed to care for you quite literally is bursting at the seams. This means less time for your doctor to learn who you are, what your health problems are, and to design a plan to diagnose and treat you. As I've alluded to in a prior chapter, the average American is taking more than one prescription medicine and is dealing with one or more chronic health problems, and many reside in underserved areas of the nation with regard to access to a doctor. So what can you do to help yourself when your doctor doesn't seem to be listening?

First, let's dig deeper into why this is so. Let's start with time and the lack of it. Doctors are under tremendous pressure to see lots of patients each day. The reasons are twofold: (1) increased numbers of sick people, and (2) complex financial factors and incentives to see more patients. Second, with the advent of the electronic medical record, doctors are often tapping away at the keyboard during your visit, which means less direct, quality time paying attention to you and your problems. Third, doctors are human, and that means they carry with them the biases and prejudices, unfortunate as they are, that the rest of us possess. Shockingly, some studies have shown that white doctors pay less attention to minority patients, particularly African Americans, and that can lead to missing a diagnosis or misdiagnosing a problem. There's no excuse for that.

So what can you do to make the most of your visit to the doctor? Assuming you've got your list of questions (and if you don't have one, make one!), here are some of my favorite tips on how to help ensure you get the answers you need:

- **Share your top two (or at most three) concerns** at the beginning of the appointment, so your doctor will know what needs to be covered. For suggestions on how to redirect the conversation when your doctor digresses, follow the next piece of advice.
- **Rehearse your questions.** You may get nervous if your doctor seems rushed. Pre-appointment prep—even if it's just in your head—will help you make your points clearly and effectively.
- **Don't diagnose yourself.** Just describe what's going on without a self-diagnosis. Otherwise, you might bias your doctor, leading to misdiagnosis.
- **Share information about yourself.** The more nonmedical information your doctor knows about you, the better he will relate to you as a person and not just a set of *symptoms*.
- **Request a response by email or a follow-up phone call** if the doctor doesn't have time during your visit to answer all of your questions. Or ask if a nurse practitioner is qualified and available to talk, or book another appointment for a consultation to finish talking things through.
- **Find out how to get follow-up questions answered.** Naturally, you may have more questions that come up after

your appointment. Does your doctor have a patient portal that can be used for such communications? Should you call the office or email your questions?

- **Bring an up-to-date list of all the medications you take.** Make sure you list not only prescription drugs, but also over-the-counter medications, herbal remedies, vitamins, and other dietary supplements. These can all react with one another. Also, list the condition for which you take each drug.
- **Include the correct name, spelling, usage, and dosage.** A warning here: Many drugs—for example, Xanax (for anxiety) and Zantac (to treat ulcers)—sound similar. A comprehensive and accurate list that includes the condition for which a drug or supplement has been prescribed will help prevent confusion and errors. This is especially important when dealing with healthcare professionals who don't speak English as their first language.
- **Inform practitioners about any drug allergies or sensitivities and all preexisting conditions.** For example, perhaps you are allergic to penicillin. While this information should appear on your chart, don't take for granted that it does. Reminding healthcare providers of your medical history, including drug allergies, is a simple and effective way to avoid potentially life-threatening medical errors.
- **Do your research.** It takes time and effort but is often worth it. If you are scheduled to take a new drug or undergo a test or procedure, first research it at reliable government, hospital, or university-based websites such as www.medlineplus.gov or www.mayoclinic.org or www.jhu.edu (Johns Hopkins). Peer-reviewed journals such as the *Journal of the American Medical Association* (jama.ama-assn.org) and the *New England Journal of Medicine* (www.nejm.org) can also be excellent sources of information. An objective nonbiased drug assessment

database is available through both print and online subscriptions (www.factsandcomparisons.com/). Ask your healthcare provider and/or pharmacist whether they use it.

- **Speak up.** Ask your doctor the right questions. Do I really need this drug/test/procedure? What are the risks versus benefits? Is this the best drug/test/procedure for my diagnosis? What about side effects? In the case of tests, are the results typically straightforward or subject to interpretation? How often is this test/procedure performed at your facility? How often does the surgeon or other medical practitioner perform it? In both cases, the more often, the better. Will there be pain or discomfort? If your physician can't or won't take the time to answer your questions, it's time to consider getting a new physician.

- **Choose a friend or family member to be your advocate.** When you're sick, it's all too easy to get nervous and forget the questions you want to ask or fail to recall your physician's advice. It's not only comforting to have a trusted advocate by your side at such times, it also contributes to a better comprehension of the situation on your part, and more accountability on the part of your caregivers. If you're in the hospital, try to have someone with you or visiting frequently so they can get help or the nurse's attention if need be.

- **Take personal responsibility.** After all, shouldn't you remain in charge of your own health? Responsibility includes not just your interactions with medical practitioners, but also making the essential lifestyle changes (I keep harping about) that reduce your risk of illness.

In the years ahead, we will continue to hear more about this important health topic. Given that "bundling" payments (third party's paying only a set amount for a certain medical scenario and no more than that) and that hospitals will now have to "eat" the costs of their medical misadventures (due to Medicare's refusal to provide coverage for "serious preventable events," with a stipulation that prevents billing patients for them), it's clear that they will focus intently on reducing these occurrences. That can only be good news. And meanwhile, Medicare's new hospital inpatient provisions will result not only in an estimated savings for the government of millions annually—but we can only hope, the saving of many lives as well.

Not as common as doctors' office visits, but all too common nonetheless, is a visit to the emergency room (ER), an event no one wants or looks forward to. ER visits, by their very nature, are of higher acuity than mere doctor's office visits and are best handled when you or a caretaker or patient advocate are prepared in advance.

In Case of Emergency: Always Carry This Health Information

Those of us of a certain age will remember a radio (and later television show called *Dragnet*), where the hardboiled detective Joe Friday would tell witnesses to alleged crimes, "All we want are the facts, ma'am." The detective, played by Jack Webb, was often short on time and full of questions, so he needed to get to the point.

When you as a patient need to go to the emergency room, and time counts, the doctors and nurses need "just the facts" to get a rapid and accurate assessment of your medical history and condition. Recently, a financial services adviser I know wanted to make a service available for his clients. The service would provide essential medical information in just such a scenario so that medical personnel can quickly assess what's important in one's medical history. I thought that was a great idea.

In light of that, I'd like to suggest the kind of information you need to share quickly and accurately, whether on a 5-by-8-inch card, a piece of paper, or some electronic device, in case of a medical emergency.

Roughly, the information falls into five basic categories: drug and food allergies, medication list, ongoing medical conditions, prior surgeries, and medical directives. Most are self-explanatory, but let's talk about each.

- **Drug and food allergies (and sensitivities) are essential to communicate to medical people.** An allergy is where you get a true anaphylactic reaction to a drug or food—where you may break out in hives, have difficulty breathing, and your windpipe swells. This is not to be confused with a sensitivity or adverse reaction, where an antibiotic might cause stomach upset. Also, food allergies, such as to shellfish, are important to know about because some intravenous contrast dyes might cause an anaphylactic reaction when given to such patients.

- **Your medication list is an important part of your medical history.** You should include all prescriptions, over-the-counter medications, and supplements on this list. This ensures that medical folks know what you are taking and what drug choices to make when treating you while you are under their care. It's also helpful to reduce the incidence of adverse drug interactions or overdose.

- **Medical conditions.** The importance of divulging your ongoing medical conditions is self-explanatory. Doctors and nurses need to know your major medical conditions, such as hypertension, diabetes, thyroid problems, cancers, autoimmune diseases, and the like. Use common sense when compiling this list; it's not essential that personnel know you once had poison ivy or an ear infection years ago.

- **Prior surgeries.** Again, use common sense. The fact that you had your appendix out is very important if you have abdominal pain. The fact that you had a small noncancerous skin lesion removed 10 years ago is not important. When in doubt, ask your doctor what to put down on your list.

- **Medical directives.** Finally, your directives regarding your "code" status (relating to heroic, lifesaving measures), your religious preferences (e.g., Jehovah's witnesses do not accept blood transfusions), whether you have a living will, your organ donor status, and the contact numbers for your primary doctor, family, and friends who are responsible for you go a long way in reducing ambiguity and confusion.

So be smart and take time to fill out these items. Carry it with you— give copies to key loved ones—and remember to review it periodically for updates. That way, when you are asked to present "just the facts," you'll be ready.

How do you protect yourself if you have to get admitted to the hospital, either emergently or electively? I have information that will be helpful. Some of this is repetitive, but still it is worth repeating.

How to Stay Safe in the Hospital: The Best Ways to Prevent Medical Errors

As many as 195,000 patients die each year in U.S. hospitals because of medical errors, according to a recent study by HealthGrades, a leading healthcare rating company. Here's how to stay safe next time you're in the hospital. If you're too incapacitated by your illness or injury to do these things for yourself, a family member can do many of them for you.

- **Keep a list of prescribed medications with dosages.** You can get this list from the attending physician (the doctor in charge of your case), an intern, resident, or nurse. Receiving the wrong medication is one of the most common—and dangerous—hospital errors. When a hospital staff member hands you a pill or starts to hook an intravenous (IV) bag to your arm, ask what you're being given. If the drug isn't on the list of medications you have been prescribed, ask "What does this treat?" If the answer isn't a condition that you think you have, double-check that the drug provider knows your name and birthday, to confirm you're the patient he/she thinks you are. Make sure it's not a drug with a similar name. If you've been prescribed Zantac and someone's trying to give you Xanax, or you take Celebrex but the nurse shows up with Cerebyx, someone may have misheard the instructions and provided the wrong medication. Also, if it is a drug you've been prescribed but you previously received a different dosage, make sure the change was intentional.

- **Label yourself.** If you're in the hospital for an operation on a limb, a lung, or anything else that you have more than one of on or in your body, use a marker or ballpoint pen to write "this arm," "this leg," or just "yes" on the side that should go under the knife, so there is no confusion in the operating room. (At some hospitals, your surgeon will sign his initials to the body part in advance of your operation.) Don't use an "X" to mark the spot, because an "X" is ambiguous—it could be misinterpreted as "not here." If you're allergic to any medications, make a sign to this effect and post it over your hospital bed. Example: "Allergic to Penicillin."

- **Schedule your hospital stay wisely.** New interns, residents, and medical school students begin assignments at teaching hospitals in early July. (In Britain, it is macabrely referred to as "Killing Wednesday," when the new doctors start their clinical careers on that day of the week.) If possible, postpone elective procedures until a different time, when young medical professionals have more experience.

- **If you can't avoid a July stay in a teaching hospital, be wary about what you let interns and medical students do.** If one wants to draw blood, insert a catheter, or perform another common hospital task, ask how many times he/she has done it before. If the answer doesn't fill you with confidence, insist that a nurse or resident take over. Also, at any time of the year, try to schedule your surgery for early in the day. By the end of a long day, even the most skilled surgeons aren't at the top of their game. Also, because patients aren't allowed to eat or drink before surgery, a late operation means extra hours of hunger, thirst, and worry.

- **Get to know the staff.** A wide range of doctors, nurses, physician's assistants, interns, residents, orderlies, and others might be involved in your care. Whenever a new face arrives, politely ask his name and what his role is, unless his name tag makes this obvious, then engage in some friendly conversation. If you make a personal connection with everyone involved in your care, it reduces the odds that you'll be mistaken for a different patient, with potentially dangerous results. It also increases the odds that you'll get prompt care. Because most hospital patients are preoccupied with their health problems, the few who remain composed, personable, and interested in the hospital staff often are treated more favorably.

- **Know who should do what.** Find out when you can expect your attending physician to visit your bedside and save any questions you have until then. Answers you receive from anyone else might not be definitive. Don't let a UAP (also known as unlicensed assistive personnel or nurse assistant) insert an IV or catheter, change a sterile dressing, give you a shot, or feed you through a tube. Such tasks should be handled by trained medical staff, such as a registered nurse. Check the person's name tag. If there's no designation, such as RN, ask what his training is.

- **Employ great effort to select the right surgeon.** Unless it is an emergency, you shouldn't necessarily settle for the first surgeon you're sent to. When you meet with a surgeon for a consultation, ask: Are you board-certified in this specialty? Or check this on the website of the American Board of Medical Specialties (www.abms.org). You will have to register, but it is free. How many times have you performed this exact procedure? You want someone who has done it hundreds or even thousands of times. If the procedure is rare, you at least want a surgeon who performs it dozens of times per year.

- **Find the right hospital.** If your surgeon has privileges at more than one hospital in your area, the annual "America's Best Hospital Guide" from *U.S. News and World Report* (https://health.usnews.com/best-hospitals) can help you decide which facility is best for a given procedure. Be aware that your health insurance might limit you to a particular hospital or restrict your choice of surgeons.

- **Plan for the unexpected before you wind up in a hospital.** Ask your doctor now which ER in your region he considers the best, assuming that there's more than one. (Of course, in situations where every second counts, the closest ER is almost always the best choice.)

- **Speak up.** Make no effort to conceal your pain in a crowded ER—the ER staff might equate a quiet patient with a low-priority medical problem and treat others ahead of you. If you must wait, let the staff know if the pain gets worse, you have trouble breathing, feel increasingly lightheaded, or lose feeling in, or control over, part of your body.

- **Encourage bedside visitors, if it is allowed.** Visitors don't just keep you company in the hospital. They can keep an eye on the quality of your care when you're unable to do so yourself. And because hospital employees know that family members keep an eye on what's going on, more visitors tend to mean more attention from the staff.

- **Warn your anesthesiologist of any loose teeth you may have.** A loose tooth could be knocked out during intubation (when a breathing tube is placed in your windpipe), causing a potentially serious infection if the tooth reaches your lungs. Also, ask your doctor about removing any dentures or artificial teeth before you're taken to the operating room.

We've talked about doctor's office visits, the increasingly common ER visit, and the all too common hospital admission, now let's focus on outpatient surgery, where most surgical interventions these days take place. How can you safeguard yourself in this instance?

Protecting Yourself During Surgery

Of the approximately 35 million annual surgeries in the United States, outpatient procedures account for at least 60% of them. Advances in pain management and surgical techniques (such as laparoscopic procedures, which require only a small incision) mean that patients who once would have spent several days in the hospital now can be discharged the same day from an outpatient facility.

Complication rates typically are usually low for these procedures, but patients can further reduce their risks—and recover faster after the surgery—by taking an active role.

In Advance

Before scheduling your procedure, be sure to do the following:

- Check out the facility. It is important that the facility where you have the procedure has a so-called crash cart—the equipment and drugs that are used for cardiac emergencies. Crash carts are mandatory in hospitals but optional in many outpatient clinics. Also important: Ask your surgeon if the facility stocks dantrolene (Dantrium). It's an antidote for malignant hyperthermia, an anesthesia-related complication that occurs only rarely but can be fatal unless dantrolene is given immediately.

- Check out the surgeon. Before scheduling a procedure, make sure that the surgeon is board-certified in that particular specialty. To find out, ask the doctor. If you are uncomfortable doing so, you could mention that you read in this book that board-certification is important and that is why you are asking. Also, make sure that the surgeon has done many of these procedures. If you're having cataract surgery, for example, someone who does 40 or 50 cataract procedures a week is likely to have better results, with fewer complications, than someone who does the procedure only occasionally.

- Review and report your medications. Your surgeon and anesthesiologist should know about every drug (and supplement) you're taking. Bring a list of your medications and supplements (and/or the bottles) when you meet with the doctor. Why this matters: You might need to adjust the doses or frequency of drugs or supplements that you're currently taking. If you have asthma, for example, the stress of surgery can cause a flare-up. You might be advised to use an inhaler prior to the procedure. Diabetics who use insulin, on the other hand, might be told to skip (or reduce) a dose before surgery. The combination of presurgical fasting and a normal dose of insulin could cause blood glucose to fall too low. In addition, some commonly used drugs and supplements, such as aspirin and ginkgo, inhibit blood clotting and can be risky when taken within several days of some procedures.

- Ask about pain control. Don't assume that your surgeon will aggressively manage pain—many do not. Uncontrolled pain releases the stress hormone cortisol, which impairs immunity and slows healing. People in pain also move around less, which increases the risk for blood clots.

In the past, surgeons mainly depended on narcotics (such as codeine) for postsurgical pain relief. These drugs are effective but may cause side effects, including urinary retention, nausea, and even itching.

Ask your surgeon (or the anesthesiologist) to discuss non-narcotic alternatives, such as nerve blocks (which can control pain for several days). One type of nerve block is the "ON-Q," which dispenses a drip of anesthetic into surgical wounds. Your surgeon can also offer patient-controlled analgesia, which allows patients to manage their own pain with the push of a button.

Pre-Surgery Planning

As you get closer to the time of the surgery, do the following:

- Stop smoking for at least 72 hours before the procedure— longer is better. Not smoking prior to surgery will improve circulation and wound healing, as well as ciliary function— the ability of hairlike projections in the lungs to remove mucus, which is important for the prevention of postsurgical pneumonia.
- Eat lightly the day before the procedure. Clear soups, rice, fruits, and vegetables are ideal. Anesthesia frequently causes

constipation. Easy-to-digest foods leave less residue in the digestive tract and help reduce postsurgical gas and cramping.
- Don't chew gum prior to surgery. It stimulates the secretion of gastric juices that can interfere with your breathing and cause choking (asphyxia) during the procedure.
- Don't shave the area that is undergoing the surgery. Even a new blade can cause thousands of invisible abrasions/nicks that can allow bacteria to enter. Shaving ahead of time gives bacteria a chance to multiply and cause an infection. If a surgical site needs to be shaved, someone on the operating team will do it right before making the incision.

After-Surgery Care

What you can do to feel better and recover faster:

- Stay warm. The blankets used in medical settings are notoriously thin. If you're cold when you wake up in the recovery room, ask for extra blankets. Patients who maintain a normal body temperature, known as normothermia, during and after surgery heal more quickly and get fewer infections than those who are cold.
- Breathe deeply and cough. The drugs used for general anesthesia can impair normal lung movements and increase the risk for pneumonia.
- Recommended: As soon as you're physically able, take deep breaths for a few minutes every hour or two. Make yourself cough, even if you don't have to. Coughing and other exaggerated respiratory movements help clear the airways. This is particularly important for those who are older, sedentary, or overweight.

- Move as soon as you can. Moving soon after a procedure reduces the risk for blood clots, improves muscle strength, and helps clear the lungs. If you can, stand up and walk. If you're not able (or allowed) to stand, move in bed. Stretch your arms and legs, roll from one side to the other, or merely flex your muscles.
- Don't put up with nausea. It is among the most frequent—and the most feared—side effects of anesthesia. Anesthesiologists now can choose from among six to eight different drugs to prevent it. If you feel sick when you wake up, tell your doctor. If one drug doesn't work, another one probably will.

Because most surgery and some procedures will require some form of anesthesia, there are things you can do here to protect yourself as well.

How Not to Be a Victim of Anesthesia Error

What do heart disease, diabetes, heartburn, and high (or low) blood pressure have in common? These are among the many conditions that can affect your reaction to anesthesia and thus your safety.

Each year, about 21 million Americans who undergo elective or emergency surgeries receive general anesthesia (a method of preventing pain by rendering a patient temporarily unconscious with drugs that are inhaled through a mask or an endotracheal tube, or that are given intravenously).

Possible complications include the following:

- **Anesthesia awareness.** According to research published in the *New England Journal of Medicine*, 1 or 2 of every 1,000 people who undergo general anesthesia "wake up" to some degree during the operation.

This so-called "awareness" may allow patients to hear conversations in the operating room while they remain immobilized and unable to speak. In rare cases—about 30,000 surgeries in the United States each year—patients also feel pain while they are unable to move or speak.

To avoid this problem, a patient's heart rate, blood pressure, breathing, and other vital signs are closely monitored during general anesthesia. About 60% of operating rooms in the United States also have bispectral index systems. These monitors record certain types of brain activity that can signal anesthesia awareness.

Among those at greatest risk: people who have low blood pressure. Because most anesthesia lowers blood pressure, people who have low blood pressure (chronic or acute, such as that due to injury-related blood loss) usually are given less anesthetic. Also at risk: heavy drinkers who tend to metabolize anesthesia more quickly than people who do not drink heavily.

Self-defense: Tell your anesthesiologist if you have low blood pressure, and be completely honest about the amount of alcohol you drink.

- **Coma, neurological damage, or death.** These devastating complications occur in about 1 in every 250,000 surgeries in which general anesthesia is used each year in the United States. The most common cause is failure of the medical team to "ventilate"—that is, provide a means for the patient to breathe.

  Among those at greatest risk: people who are obese—being overweight can cause obstruction of the airway, including the throat and larynx; those who have had prior surgery or radiation of the neck, mouth, or airway—surgery or radiation to these areas can stiffen the tissues in the neck and mouth, making it more difficult to ventilate the patient; anyone with sleep apnea (temporary cessation of breathing during sleep); persons with a history of difficulty when being intubated (insertion of a tube to keep the airway open) during past surgeries.

Self-defense: Tell your anesthesiologist if any of these risk factors apply to you. Even if you've never been diagnosed with sleep apnea, let him/her know if you snore at night or feel unusually tired during the day. These can be signs of sleep apnea, which obstructs the airway.

- **Pneumonia.** Thousands of Americans develop anesthesia-related pneumonia each year. One of the most common causes is the backup (reflux) of stomach acid, which can be inhaled (aspirated) into the lungs while a patient is under anesthesia, leading to pneumonia.

  Among those at greatest risk: People who have chronic heartburn (known as gastroesophageal reflux disease, or GERD) or a hiatal hernia (in which the stomach passes partly or completely into the chest cavity)—both conditions make patients prone to aspiration, and those who are obese, have diabetes, or have diseases of the nervous system, such as Parkinson's disease. Obesity, diabetes, and nervous system disorders increase the risk for aspiration because they can delay emptying of stomach contents.

  Self-defense: Your anesthesiologist may not ask about heartburn or hiatal hernias, but it's important to tell him if you are affected by these conditions. If you do have GERD, drugs that reduce stomach acid, such as lansoprazole (Prevacid) or ranitidine (Zantac), may be prescribed.

  Important: Carefully follow your hospital's guidelines on food and liquid intake before surgery.

- **Heart attack or stroke.** Each year, about 1 in 10,000 patients suffer heart attack or stroke while under anesthesia.

  Among those at greatest risk: people with high blood pressure (140/90 or above) and/or heart disease. A history of high blood pressure can increase a patient's risk for stroke because of accompanying blood vessel changes, such as stiffening of the arteries. Heart disease often causes a thickening of the arteries to the heart that can lead to cardiovascular complications during anesthesia, resulting in a heart attack.

  Self-defense: Inform your anesthesiologist if you have high blood pressure or heart disease.

Getting the Best Care

Most surgical patients do not meet the anesthesiologist until moments before surgery. If possible, ask your surgeon beforehand who will be administering the anesthetic and whether you can meet with him a day or two before the surgery so he has more time to review your medical history and address any of your concerns.

Tell your anesthesiologist if:

- **You take any medications or supplements.** Blood pressure, diabetes, and blood-thinning drugs are among those that may need to be discontinued prior to surgery. Speak to your surgeon for specific instructions. Herbal remedies, including St. John's wort and garlic, may need to be discontinued before the operation because they may interact with the anesthetic.
- **Anyone in your family has ever had a bad reaction to general anesthesia, such as delayed awakening.** In some cases, bad reactions to anesthesia may be genetic.

And one final word of caution:

Don't Let What Happened to Joan Rivers Happen to You: Additional Ways to Make Outpatient Surgery Safer

Ever since Joan Rivers died after a routine surgical procedure at an outpatient center in Manhattan, people have been wondering if they're better off having surgery in a hospital. The reality is that the vast majority of outpatient procedures go off without a hitch. But you can reduce your risk by getting involved before the procedure. These are important steps.

Know Your Physical Status

Ask your doctor about your "physical status classification." The American Society of Anesthesiologists uses a numerical scale to assess a patient's surgical risks. Patients with higher physical status (PS) scores (four or five) because of health problems should have procedures done in hospitals because their risk for complications is higher.

Example: A patient who needs a knee replacement also might have poorly controlled diabetes, kidney insufficiency, and nerve damage. His/her PS might be rated as four—too high to safely have a major procedure at an outpatient center.

In general, patients with PS scores of one through three—with one being generally healthy and three indicating that they have serious diseases that aren't life-threatening—are good candidates for outpatient procedures.

Pick Your Surgeon Carefully

Don't assume that every surgeon in an outpatient center has the same experience—or the same credentials.

Suppose you're planning to get Botox or Restylane injections. These are not as simple as most people think. For the best results—and the lowest risk for complications—you should have the procedure done by a physician who is board-certified in plastic and reconstructive surgery.

Caution: In many states, many procedures can be done by any physician who has undergone minimal training in these procedures, such as a weekend course or three-day seminar. These doctors might be board-certified in something, but not necessarily in the field that concerns you.

Also important: The amount of experience. Studies have clearly shown that doctors who do a lot of procedures have better results, with fewer complications, than those who do them less often.

Example: If I were planning to have LASIK eye surgery, I wouldn't feel comfortable seeing a surgeon who had done the procedure 50 times. I would want someone whose total cases numbered in the hundreds or even thousands.

Insist on Pain Control

Most people assume that their surgeons will do everything possible to minimize postoperative pain. Not true. Some doctors are reluctant to order strong painkillers on an ongoing basis because they worry that the patient will become addicted. Or they mainly use narcotics (opioids, such as codeine and morphine) that dull the pain but can cause unpleasant and sometimes dangerous side effects, including impaired breathing, constipation, itching, nausea, and vomiting.

Although I cover pain in more detail in Chapter 4, it is wise to note that poorly controlled pain is among the most serious postoperative complications. It impairs immunity and increases the risk for infection, it slows healing times, and it can increase the risk for blood clots when patients hurt too much to move normally.

My advice: Tell your surgeon that you're terrified of pain. Ask what he/she plans to use to relieve your pain—and emphasize that you would like to avoid narcotics if at all possible.

Also, ask about bupivacaine (Exparel), a nonnarcotic anesthetic that was recently approved by the FDA. The active ingredient is encapsulated in liposomal (fat-based) particles and slowly released over 72 hours. When injected into the surgical area, it relieves pain as effectively as narcotics, with fewer side effects. (I will discuss the benefits of Exparel and other innovative methods of pain control in a later chapter.)

Beware of Using Supplements During Surgery and Anesthesia

Tell your doctor about everything you're taking. Surgeons and anesthesiologists routinely ask patients about medications they're using. They don't always think to ask about supplements.

This is a dangerous oversight because many supplements—along with garden-variety over-the-counter medications such as aspirin—can interact with the drugs used during and after surgery.

Examples: Garlic supplements increase the risk for excessive bleeding, particularly when they're combined with aspirin. The herbs ephedra and kava can interfere with anesthetics.

Patients who are taking natural remedies—including vitamin E, echinacea, ginseng, valerian, and St. John's wort—should ask their doctors if they need to quit taking them. You may need to stop two weeks or more before the procedure. Aspirin should be discontinued two to three days before.

Can They Plan for the Worst at This Facility?

Even routine procedures sometimes go south. Most outpatient surgical centers are equipped with crash carts (used for cardiac emergencies) and other equipment and drugs for handling serious complications—but some don't have these on hand.

Ask the surgeon if a crash cart will be available. Also ask the following:

- Is there dantrolene (Dantrium)? It can reverse a rare but deadly complication from anesthesia known as malignant hyperthermia. The drug is always stocked in hospitals, but an outpatient center might not have it.
- Is there succinylcholine (Anectine, Quelicin)? It's a fast-acting paralytic agent that assists doctors in quickly intubating patients who can't breathe—one of the most dangerous complications of anesthesia. It has been reported that Joan Rivers might have lived if this drug had been available.

Don't Put Up with Nausea

It is estimated that 30% of all postsurgical patients will experience nausea, retching, or vomiting. These are among the most common surgical complications.

My advice: Tell your anesthesiologist/surgeon if you've suffered from surgery-related nausea in the past. He/she can administer granisetron (Kytril) or ondansetron (Zofran), which helps prevent nausea in most patients.

Also, consider buying a Reliefband, a device you wear on your wrist that sends electrical impulses to the nausea center in your brainstem to tell it to "quiet down." Visit reliefband.com for more information and to purchase one.

Get Moving

Try to get moving as soon as you can. Surgeons formerly recommended lengthy bed rest for postsurgical patients. They now know that it's better to move around as soon as possible to prevent constipation, urinary retention, and muscle weakness, among other common complications.

As soon as you're able, get up and walk (with your doctor's permission, of course). If you can't stand right away, at least move in bed. Stretch your legs. Move your arms. Roll over, sit up, and so on. Any kind of physical movement increases blood flow and improves recovery times. It also improves the movement of your lungs, which can help prevent postsurgical pneumonia.

Stem Cell Clinics Can Dispense Dangerous Medicine

One additional growing, but often unregulated, area of medical care to be mindful of and cautious about is stem cell therapy. Two large reports in the *Washington Post* a few years back have reported the dangers to patients posed by practitioners at stem cell clinics. These clinics, some of which are largely unregulated and independent, have been involved in various forms of litigation, ranging from lawsuits over medical malpractice, product liability, and lack of sterile products and procedures. One particularly blatant suit described how a woman was supposedly treated for macular degeneration with injections of her own reprocessed adipose tissue into her eyes. The result has almost left her completely blind.

The FDA and other regulatory agencies have been remiss in regulating this widely growing area of medicine. Some regulators and observers have gone so far as to say that some practices border on human experimentation. Indeed, the *Post* article quoted Charles Murray, director of the Institute for Stem Cell and Regenerative Medicine at the University of Washington as saying, "We're afraid that these charlatans will besmirch the reputation of legitimate work we have spent decades trying to bring to the clinic."

In theory, clinic operators say treatments work like this: Fat tissue is extracted from the patient, and physical and chemical processing refines down the material to isolate stem cells, which is then injected back into the patient in certain problem target areas. But stem cell researchers refute this type of elementary process, saying in criticism that the material extracted contains little-to-no stem cells and that this reinjected material does not do the regenerative work purported. Also, the FDA notes that few stem cell therapies have been approved, with products derived from umbilical cord and placental blood. These therapies are most promising in leukemia and other blood diseases.

Many stem cell clinics have opened claiming to treat conditions as diverse as heart disease, Parkinson's, stroke, vision problems, arthritis, autism, and more. But Timothy Caufield, a health law professor at University of Alberta (Canada) said in the *Post* article: "What they're really selling is false hope . . . they're taking a legitimate and developing field of science and using it to prey on patients who are desperate for a cure."

And the "false hope" they are selling can be quite expensive. Insurance seldom covers this type of "care," and patients can pay large sums out of pocket. So large that the people peddling this can make big money, money that they've attempted to woo me with. In my recent professional life, I have received multiple offers of high-paying and even partnership arrangements by these types of clinics. I did my research, looked at what they were doing, and turned each one down. For various reasons, including the personalities of the principals, the procedures performed and the ancillary quasi-medical marketing being offered (supplements and pain therapies of unproven value and more). The setup just didn't pass the sniff-test.

Since reports of patients being blinded have emerged, the FDA finally acted to stop two companies involved in alleged stem cell therapy: the U.S. Stem Cell Clinic and the Cell Surgical Network. Both companies disagree with the ruling and one has vowed to fight it. But the more than 700 stem cell clinics across the country may now come under closer scrutiny since Leigh Turner, a bioethicist at the University of Minnesota, described the two previously mentioned companies in another *Washington Post* article as "the most notorious in the industry for marketing unproven treatments for incurable diseases."

My advice to you: Steer clear of all freestanding, non-university or non-medical-school-affiliated clinics hawking these treatments. Until the FDA and scientific literature prove the efficacy and safety of these procedures, I'd exercise caution. These treatments are very much revenue-driven and can be very expensive. We've already seen scores of patients being hurt. Don't be one of them.

Also, a final word of caution: The latest technology is not always better. It can be as true in the operating room as in the cockpit of the most advanced aircraft.

Aviation, Medicine, and Other Potential Technology Disasters

Sadly, relatively recent world news has fixated on the disastrous second crash in five months of a Boeing 737 Max aircraft, a plane that was supposed to be the pinnacle of performance, technology, and even safety. The plane, an Ethiopian Airways jet (owned by the same airline I flew in the summer of 2018 to a medical mission in

Tanzania), was lost shortly after takeoff on March 10, 2019, killing all 157 people aboard. Boeing has insisted the plane is safe and that the crashes had nothing to do with defects in the plane. Owners of the plane are skeptical, however, leading many airlines in nations, including (after a conspicuous and controversial delay) the United States, to ground their fleet of 737 Max's until the question of safety and/or defects is resolved.

The FBI is currently involved in a potential criminal probe of Boeing, related to whether the company had knowledge of the software defect that is believed to have led to the crashes. There have also been recent stories of "jump seat" pilots having to take over for perplexed and panicked pilots who were not trained, briefed, or otherwise skilled to handle this seemingly prevalent flaw that kept turning the plane's nose down.

How does any of this apply to medical practice and patients, you might ask? Easy—it concerns technology and the increasingly limited role of human operator control. There have long been comparisons made between aviation safety and medical safety, particularly in the areas of anesthesia and surgery. Indeed, in my own specialty of anesthesiology, inducing anesthesia has often been compared to "takeoff," and emergence from it has been likened to "landing" the patient. What happens between those events has often been compared to maintaining stability, avoiding turbulence, and keeping the ride (and anesthetic course) smooth.

But as companies who make planes, anesthesia equipment, surgical equipment, and self-driving cars (who have had their share of injuries and even deaths) might not want to admit, this move away from operator control toward automation—often showcased to drive profits with technologic glitz and sexiness—might turn out to be a dangerous one. This is nowhere more evident than in this entry from the front page of the *Washington Post* on March 12, 2019, where reporters Aaron Gregg and Christian Davenport write:

The crash . . . puts the spotlight on Boeing, which already faced scrutiny for its October crash in Indonesia and concerns that a software update to the 737 could make it hard to override a malfunctioning autopilot system when it steers the plane into a nosedive.

It is this possible inability to override that reminded me of personal experience with some anesthesia and surgical equipment that has, in the past, caused or could have caused patient harm. I recall one case where a woman was undergoing a hysteroscopy, where fluid is flushed in the uterus to help visualize the female reproductive tract with an endoscope. Everyone was paying attention to the screen where the interior of the uterus was visible, but no one was really paying attention to the patient. Instead, an alarm system that kept going off due to imbalances in fluid-in versus fluid-out of the patient occupied much of the staff's attention and efforts. Repeated fiddling with warning sounds controls and real-time trouble-shooting of the equipment took up valuable attention that should have been placed on the patient instead, whose lungs were rapidly filling with fluid due to a severe fluid imbalance caused by a faulty input to the monitor. The patient went into severe congestive heart failure and required a tracheostomy (cutting a breathing hole in her neck to her trachea) because of an inability to intubate her (which involves inserting a breathing tube down the windpipe). Eventually the crisis was resolved, but it was a close call.

Touching on a similar subject, I remember when laparoscopic gallbladder removal first emerged in the early 1990s. Prior to that, gallbladders were removed with a large, open incision in the upper abdomen. The learning curve to skillfully operate the laparoscopy equipment for abdominal surgery required extra time, effort, and attention by the surgeon. Bells and whistles went off like crazy, as pressure gauges, electrocautery connections, and gas supply meters to insufflate (blow gas into) the abdomen all needed attention. This took critical attention away from the patient and onto the equipment. The very technology that was supposed to help patients instead, at least in the learning phase of practice, ended up putting the patient at risk. Not only that, but as surgeons came to rely on laparoscopic gallbladder removal as the primary method, they lost their skills in the old method, a method that sometimes they might have to fall back on in case the laparoscopic technique failed. Many newer surgeons are not even adequately trained in the older method.

The point of this discussion is that, in medicine, as in aviation, more technology and fancier equipment may not always be better. In fact, anything that diminishes human operator control, flawed as that might be, might actually be more dangerous than previously thought. The same *Post* article concluded by saying:

> the controversy revived an ongoing debate about what degree of automation is safest for airplanes—and how much human pilots should maintain.

So what can you, the patient, do to protect yourself? Unfortunately, not a lot, short of telling your medical team, "Remember me and pay close attention to me, not just to your equipment!"

What really needs to happen is that both the medical and aviation industries, as well as any industry entrusted with public safety, ensure that skilled operators are well-versed in the use and design of their equipment, have the ability to understand and override faulty warning systems, and most important, are able to devote their primary attention to what they were trained to do, whether that's wielding a scalpel, steering clear of turbulence, or landing a multi-ton plane full of hundreds of people safely. After all, pilots, doctors, and even cab drivers were meant and trained to do a job with their heads and their hands, not troubleshoot overly complex systems that might well have been designed to make the product used appear to be more sophisticated, modern, and appealing.

CHAPTER 4

Pain

The Universal Scourge

In 2018, Bridget Kuehn, writing in the article "Chronic Pain Prevalence" in the *Journal of the American Medical Association* reviewed the CDC's statistics for 2016 regarding pain in America. The conclusions drawn were that 20% of Americans had chronic pain in 2016 and 8% suffered what is called "high-impact" chronic pain, defined as pain "limiting life or work activities on most days or every day during the past 6 months."

We've all heard too much about the opioid crisis in our country and the toll it has taken, both personal and financial, on people at all levels of the social strata. But if pain, whether chronic or acute, is such an issue in our society, how is it treated effectively without suffering the pitfalls inherent in its alleviation? I hope to give you some answers here.

First, a brief background. In the 1990s and the decade that followed, there was a big push in the medical community to aggressively tackle the so-called fifth vital sign: pain. A confluence of factors, including social and political pressure, pharmaceutical company marketing, and even what I call "medical political-correctness," stoked the attitude that pain after surgery, during cancer treatment, and in a variety of other clinical settings was to be avoided at all costs. In essence, the perception of pain was borderline deemed to be unacceptable. The end result of this was a massive effort to attack the problem from different angles, and one of those angles involved the increased prescribing of opiate and opiate-type medications. This had a strong hand in creating the crisis we see today.

The damage created by the opioid crisis is well-documented and is not my focus here. Instead, I'd like to highlight some newer and more innovative ways to handle pain, particularly the acute type experienced after surgery and procedures. I'll also touch on drug-free ways to ease of chronic pain.

Pain Relief Without the Pitfalls

Pain . . . we've all had it. None of us (except those who are masochists) like it or want it. From the mildest headache to the most excruciating kidney stone, pain comes in many forms and severity. It is estimated, as I've said, that 20% of Americans suffer some form of chronic pain, and when you add to this the number of us who suffer from acute pain (injuries, postsurgical pain, the common headache or toothache, etc.), it is easy to appreciate the magnitude of this problem.

Whenever possible, we all want and expect relief from pain, but few of us appreciate the potential dangers inherent in the way moderate-to-severe pain has been handled by the medical community in the last few decades. For pain that is moderate to severe—from whatever cause—there had been a prevailing view that brief, controlled use of narcotic medications such as Percocet (oxycodone) or Vicodin (hydrocodone) was acceptable and appropriate. However, in light of recent studies and literature to the contrary, we now know that these medications and those similar to them have a far wider potential for abuse, danger, and overdose than originally thought.

First, some basic physiology. The human body contains untold receptors in the central and peripheral nervous system that react to a class of naturally occurring and synthetic drugs used to relieve pain. These opiates and opioid-type medicines, as opposed to the commonly known anti-inflammatory pain medicines (aspirin, ibuprofen, naproxen, etc.), interact with these receptors to cause a decrease in pain perception and an overall feeling of well-being. However, these medications not only cause side effects, including itching, constipation, slowed breathing, and difficulty urinating to name a few, but they have the potential for addiction and tolerance (increasing doses are needed to achieve the desired pain-relieving effect). As a result, it is estimated by the National Institutes of Health (NIH) that more than two million people in our country have become addicted to this class of medication after receiving prescriptions written to relieve pain. Alarmingly high rates of near-overdoses and overdose-related deaths are reaching the hundreds of thousands each year. The government is trying to tackle the problem of addiction in new and novel ways, but the end is nowhere in sight.

What can you, the average patient who wants relief from moderate-to-severe pain, do to get the pain in check without the inherent dangers of opioid therapy? I have a few suggestions:

- When it comes to postsurgical pain, consider skipping this class of medicine altogether. Now, this won't always be possible because of the severity of some types of pain. It is up to you to decide your own tolerance for pain and how to deal with it. Consider asking your doctor for the newer injectable forms of the standard anti-inflammatory painkillers. Ibuprofen and naproxen now are available in injectable forms (another med in this class, injectable ketorolac, has been around for decades). These medicines may be appropriate in some cases to give you the pain relief you need.

- Consider the newer form of injectable acetaminophen, better known as Tylenol. Ofirmev is the brand name of this newer agent and it has shown promise for postsurgical pain relief. Realize, though, that this drug will not have the anti-inflammatory properties of the others mentioned earlier.
- A groundbreaking time-released form of the local anesthetic Exparel, mentioned in a prior chapter, has emerged as a novel way to treat surgical pain. This medication, injected by the surgeon or anesthesia provider, can result in longer-lasting pain relief with much fewer side effects compared to the nonsteroidal anti-inflammatories or narcotic medicines. I'll speak more on this in the next section.
- Alternative pain relief can be achieved with the use of specific nerve blocks. Ask the anesthesia provider if this is possible. Local anesthetics can be released over time in epidurals and other nerve blocks (for the arm, hand, leg, or foot, etc.) with the use of infusion pumps and other devices.
- Guided imagery and other modalities (neurofeedback, using brain imaging technology) are showing some promise.
- The use of medical marijuana is also gaining some traction for pain relief in some areas of the country. I'll explore this in more detail as well.

Because of the addiction and abuse problem of narcotic pain medicines, the pendulum is starting to swing away from their automatic use and toward a more cautious approach. The root causes of the epidemic have been identified—cavalier prescribing, social acceptance, and drug-company marketing efforts let the opiate genie out of the bottle decades ago. Getting the genie back in the bottle is going to be a struggle. Along with the alternative therapies I have mentioned, drug makers are now looking at painkilling medicines that have less potential for addiction and tolerance. Also, drugs like

Lyrica and Neurontin have emerged as useful players in relieving some forms of chronic pain. Today, the world of pain relief has never seen such concentrated research and innovation.

And What About Exparel, the Game-Changer?

Every so often in science, particularly in medicine, there are game-changers—innovations that are so significant and monumental that their impact affects millions of people for the better. The major game-changers can save lives. Examples might be the discovery of antibiotics, the invention of CAT scans and MRIs, and the synthesis of antiviral medicines.

Minor game-changers can be thought of as those that improve our lives, such as the development of midazolam as a safe and reliable presurgical sedative drug and the advent of propofol as a consistent and effective sleep-inducing agent for sedation and general anesthesia.

And now, a medication that falls somewhere between the major and minor game-changers, Exparel (bupivacaine liposome injectable suspension). Why is Exparel so relevant and important today?

We've all discussed the ever-present and seemingly growing opiate and opioid epidemic that is killing thousands worldwide. In the United States, a recent report by the IQVIA Institute for Human Data Science revealed these sobering facts:

- Patients across seven commonly performed surgeries were prescribed an average of 82 opioid pills to manage pain.
- Nearly 9% of surgical patients in 2017 became new persistent opioid users.
- Persistent opioid use has spiked among females, especially in women ages 18 to 34. Women are 40% more likely to become new persistent opioid users after surgery than men.

- Enough opioids were prescribed in 2017 to give every American 32 pills.
- Overdose deaths from opioids increased from 21,000 in 2010 to 50,000 in 2017. Nearly one-third of Americans say that they know someone addicted to opioids.

Enter the game-changer in pain management. Exparel is a newer medication whose application is unique and much needed. It is an injectable liquid containing microscopic fat globules called liposomes, each containing quanta (or packets) of the well-known local anesthetic bupivacaine. Bupivacaine has been around for decades, and has been used by surgeons, anesthesiologists, and pain doctors to relieve pain after all forms of surgery and to perform surgery and procedures under local anesthesia.

The people who make Exparel have figured out a way to administer bupivacaine in a safe and effective time-released formulation so that longer-term pain relief from surgical procedures can be accomplished. After it is injected by the surgeon or anesthesiologist, Exparel's tiny liposomal (fat) globules dissolve gradually over many hours, even days, releasing the local anesthetic bupivacaine into the tissues. This means that, for many patients (and I have seen this firsthand), there appears to be little or no need for any narcotic medicine to be given or taken for many days following surgery. None! That means less exposure to the addiction-risking oral opioids, fewer side effects from opioids (the most common being respiratory depression, constipation, itching, urinary retention, and hives) and fewer pain pills lying around that could be diverted (think teens, friends, and thieves) for illicit use.

To me, this is clearly a game-changer. It's perhaps not the magnitude of a penicillin-discovery game changer, but it's a breakthrough nonetheless.

Is Exparel perfect? No, no drug is perfect. Side effects, which are not frequent, include blurred vision, dizziness, nausea and constipation, among others. But generally, Exparel is very well-tolerated. When used correctly, the chance of major or even complete pain relief in the first few days following surgery is quite high. It cannot be used for all surgeries, so your doctor needs to inform you if the procedure you're having is amenable to Exparel therapy. However, I have personally seen what Exparel can do. It is truly amazing. A close friend from my anesthesia residency had a hip replacement last year and was injected with Exparel. The result? He was totally pain free for 72 hours after the surgery and did not need a single narcotic pill in that time.

That is what I call game-changing.

While I am clearly impressed by the benefits of this new pain-fighting agent, be mindful that not all surgical facilities will offer it, at least not yet.

Is There Drug-Free Postsurgical Pain Relief?

I've just described Exparel as an injectable pain medicine that reduced or eliminated the need for narcotic medications after surgery. Now, I will focus on another modality that deals not only with pain relief, but with anxiety, depression, insomnia, and even opiate withdrawal. Sound like a too-tall order? Read on.

A company called Innovative Health Solutions has designed and gotten FDA approval for a drug-free device called the BRIDGE to relieve postsurgical pain. Depending on the patient's response, it can reduce or eliminate the need for pain meds of any kind, but the main goal is to avoid opiates.

Worn for up to five days on and behind the ear, it generates electrical impulses from the outer ear to the central nervous system—to the part of the brain that partially controls stress, emotion, anxiety, depression, cravings, and pain perception. This system, the limbic system, is run by a small brain structure called the amygdala (Latin for almond). The signals sent to this area (by use of peripheral nerve field stimulation, or PNFS) have beneficial effects outside the surgical arena, as proven in some human and animal studies, as well as in research or scientific modeling. These include:

- Less perception of pain after surgery
- Less anxiety in anxious people
- Decreased depression
- Decreased insomnia
- Decreased opioid craving in people undergoing narcotic withdrawal

The device takes about 15 minutes to apply. The generator, about the size of a standard hearing aid, is housed behind the ear with tape and is connected by four small wires to electrodes implanted with tiny spikes in the skin of the ear (inserted on the ear's front, back, earlobe, and anterior to the tragus—the small cartilage flap at the front of the ear opening). Once in place, the unit generates electrical signals to the brain to achieve the desired positive effects. Side effects include mild discomfort, the potential for infection, and bleeding. After five days, the unit is removed and discarded in a sharps container.

Not all insurers cover the purchase and use of the BRIDGE, and certainly not all medical centers and doctors' offices are carrying it. The system is really in its infancy, and more studies need to be done to further prove its utility and benefits. But at a time when opioids are killing thousands of Americans each year, and prescriptions for anxiety-, depression-, and insomnia-related medications continue to skyrocket, any nonpharmacologic tool that has minimal side effects is worth a look.

Auricular acupuncture has been around for centuries, and this "shocking" twist on an old medical discipline just might be the charge many patients are seeking.

Is There New Hope for Fibromyalgia Sufferers?

There is a pain-related disease whose very existence is questioned today by many in the medical field. That condition is fibromyalgia—a diagnosis that is one of "exclusion." That is, up until recently, there was no objective test or marker for the condition. Now, a California doctor claims that has changed.

Fibromyalgia as a disease and diagnosis has been around for decades. But many doctors, even today, don't believe it exists. Characterized by any combination of muscle and joint aches, sleep disturbance, headaches, "brain fog," anxiety, depression, migraines, and irritable bowels, this condition was often dismissed as a bogus diagnosis. There was never, until today, any lab test or other medical study that could confirm its presence. For those who do believe it is real, it seems to afflict 1 out of 12 women and 1 out of 20 men. Children can even be affected.

Long the domain of rheumatologists, psychiatrists, and internists, the condition confounds patients and caregivers alike. It has been estimated that the average time until correct diagnosis is 3 to 5 years, and the average patient will have spent between $4,800 and $9,300 healthcare dollars in getting the right diagnosis. Many patients fear being labeled hypochondriacs and malingerers, and doctors who don't know much about the condition and how to treat it have been frustrated when its signs and symptoms present themselves.

All that may be changing. Dr. Bruce Gillis, a California doctor and researcher, in conjunction with the University of Illinois/ Chicago and the Harvard School of Public Health, has been examining the issue. He and his research team claim to have designed a test specific for fibromyalgia—the FM/a test—which is said to measure certain chemicals from white blood cells called mononuclear cells. The chemicals, called cytokines and chemokines, are supposed to react a certain way in the normal state of health. The test sees if these chemicals are altered in their function in a specific way indicative of fibromyalgia.

Not all insurance companies will cover the cost of the test. Also, there have been critics who say that because Dr. Gillis has a financial stake in the company (he's the CEO of EpicGenetics, the company selling the test), the test should be regarded with caution. However, because there appears to have been no major breakthroughs in diagnosing the disease, an investigation into these claims is certainly warranted. You can learn more about the test at thefmtest.com.

Concurrent with the test has been the discovery that an old TB medication, BCG, has shown promise in treating patients with fibromyalgia. I would encourage anyone who is suspected of having the condition to do the necessary research and ask your doctor if he/she is aware of this information (including an upcoming clinical trial on BCG). For a disease that has been so mysterious and elusive these many years, perhaps there is a game-changing diagnostic test and treatment on the horizon. But as I said: read, learn, and talk. This may be the most promising news about fibromyalgia to come along in years.

Healthcare Is Going to Pot

Almost every consumer of health services today has heard that medical marijuana is in clinical use. Indeed, over two dozen states and the District of Columbia now have laws on the books that allow for the use of marijuana for medicinal purposes. Incredibly, these state laws are still in violation of federal law, but for now, the U.S. government has decided to look the other way. The federal government's policy of not prosecuting states that allow for medical marijuana might cause one to think that there must be some benefit to the use of this controversial agent. But first, a little history.

Marijuana, or cannabis (as it is commonly called), has been used as a medicine for a variety of purposes for thousands of years. The ancient cultures of China, Egypt, Greece, and certain Arab populations used it for anything from wound healing to hemorrhoids to insomnia and anxiety. It is actually one of the 50 essential plants used in traditional Chinese medicine. Until the advent of aspirin and the wider use of both naturally occurring and synthetically made narcotics (opiates and opioids), marijuana enjoyed some degree of notoriety in the medical community. It wasn't until its criminalization in the United States in the twentieth century that marijuana use for medical and recreational purposes went underground. However, with opiate addiction and a growing populace of older and sicker people, scientists have turned in recent decades to the potential benefits of this most interesting of plants.

The science of marijuana as medicine can be plainly put. Our bodies contain billions of natural receptors that are stimulated by the many chemicals in marijuana that cause a number of beneficial and not-so-beneficial effects. Two of these chemicals, tetrahydrocannabinol (THC, the mind-altering component) and cannabinol (CBD, the major therapeutic part) are what we are concerned with most in discussing pot as medicine. Scientists have been able to alter the ratio of these chemicals in medical marijuana, whether in pill, vapor, tincture, edible, or dermal patch formulations, to best affect a number of medical conditions. So far, medical marijuana shows promise in:

- Reducing eye pressure in glaucoma
- Improving appetite in cancer and patients with HIV
- People who have chronic pain from a variety of causes
- Limb spasticity in patients with multiple sclerosis and other neurologic diseases

- Children with uncontrolled seizures
- Reducing nausea and vomiting in patients receiving chemotherapy
- Helping people with insomnia to sleep better
- Relieving pain in patients with rheumatoid arthritis

There are a number of other applications that are actively being studied. They include using marijuana in the treatment for cancer, diabetes, asthma, fibromyalgia, chronic fatigue, depression, PTSD, Tourette's syndrome, Crohn's disease, and many other illnesses. This truly is an exciting time in medical marijuana research.

Bear in mind there are some side effects from the use of medical marijuana, but they are usually mild. Most often they are:

- Dizziness
- Feeling tired
- Hallucinations
- Drowsiness
- Vomiting

So if you live in a state that has a medical marijuana program, I have the following suggestions:

- Do research on the web about your state's medical marijuana program, or simply call your state's board of health or medicine.
- Always deal with a reputable and licensed physician and dispensary. Do research on the internet or ask to see licenses or certificates from the state to verify compliance.
- Ask friends or relatives if they have experience with a certain provider of medical marijuana services.

- Ask your personal physician if he/she knows of a licensed marijuana practitioner. Ask if other patients have benefitted from such a regimen.
- Contact your local university medical center (if there is one in your community) to see if they have a medical marijuana program or do cannabis research.

Medical marijuana may not be for everyone. It is not a cure-all. It still, unfortunately, carries the stigma that "pot" has had for decades, even centuries. However, if you have tried other therapies for your medical issue and they have failed or you can't tolerate the side effects, strongly consider trying this most fascinating and potentially beneficial of plants. You might be pleasantly surprised.

CHAPTER 5

Pressing Issues

Public Policy, Patient Responsibility, Health Trends, and the Law

I n the Preface to this book, I briefly mentioned how I became acquainted with Bottom Line Incorporated's publications and how our common goal of helping their readers think differently and better about medicine and health were served by my blogging. In this chapter, I hope to explore a representative sampling of diverse topics that I contend are not discussed enough in mainstream media. In this chapter, unlike the others in this book, there is no unifying theme—and that is on purpose. I have curated these small articles not only to get you to think and act on their content but to pique your interest into discovering more about the important issues that may affect you personally. It is fair to say that some of the information in this chapter could even save your life or the life of someone you care about.

Healthcare and medicine, like life itself, move too quickly these days. New healthcare policies come at us from the federal government, the states themselves, and from private insurers and health plans, who must continuously keep abreast of the ever-changing laws and regulations handed down by an overly bloated system. It is truly a wonder that patients can successfully navigate the health-care system at all, let alone thrive in it. Third-party payors, Medicare, Medicaid, deductibles, health savings accounts, preauthorization, healthcare exchanges, payment bundling, big data—who under-stands and has time for all this? In my father's heyday of practice, one went to the doctor and paid cash. Then insurance companies got involved and paid a portion of the balance that was owed. Specialists and other medical professionals dedicated to your care got paid on a fee-for-service basis, which was for a long time the model for phy-sician reimbursement.

But then the government, through data collected by its entitle-ment programs and other sources, led the charge to hold down costs, with private insurers looking on. Payment bundling, where a set fee for a set clinical circumstance was doled out, is becoming more and more the payment model of choice. Ms. Jones's gallbladder removal would merit, say, $25,000 and no more, to be split up among all the doctors and institutions involved in her care. And if Ms. Jones got a lung or urinary infection or other complication during her hospi-talization, too bad. Whoever made the mistakes or appeared to offer substandard care is irrelevant: They will be forced to "eat" the excess charge. This model was and is designed, purportedly, to drive quality in outcomes. Perhaps. But what it does do is drive payment recipi-ents crazy, because many of the variables that Ms. Jones might bring to the table, like her weight, overall health, and other factors, impact how she might do in her recovery period.

Treatments, whether they be medication, new therapeutic devices, or new therapeutic approaches, are changing quickly as well. In many cases, that is good news and patients are reaping the ben-efits. One great example is the virtual "curing" of sickle cell disease, through gene therapy, as reported recently on the popular TV pro-gram *60 Minutes*.

Let's examine some of these changes, trends, innovations, and developments, some of which you might be familiar with. Perhaps others will surprise you.

To start, let's talk about men, and their all too common aversion to seeking help. Just as men are often jokingly said to be resistant to looking at a roadmap when they're lost, the same goes for when it comes to seeing the doctor.

Men: Time to "Man Up!"

Today, gender issues are in the spotlight more than ever, and men still don't go to the doctor as often as they should. Why is it that men are so stubborn about taking care of themselves?

Relatively recent articles put out by the *Huffington Post* and the American Heart Association have focused on the reasons why. The former publication has pointed out that men die earlier than women and are more likely to die from the top ten causes of death in the United States. (These are, according to the CDC: heart disease, cancer, lung disease, accidents, stroke, Alzheimer's, diabetes, flu and pneumonia, kidney disease, and suicide.) Part of this, they say, may be due to men taking more risks than women, as well as smoking and drinking to excess more than women. Men's relative social isolation and more dangerous jobs also put them at risk for earlier death. However, as foolish as some of these seem, the *Huffington Post*'s major reasons why men avoid the MD were:

- "Too busy to go"
- Fear of finding out bad news
- Discomfort of examination (prostate, rectal, etc.)
- The doctor's "personal" questions
- Getting weighed

Do visits to the doctor really save lives? You bet. Blood pressure screening, blood sugar tests, and skin and testicular examinations are but a few of the easy interventions that can prevent or help treat diseases before they have gone too far. Lifestyle changes, medical and surgical therapies, as well as psychiatric counseling can literally save lives. But symptoms have to be heard and signs of disease have to be seen to be recognized and treated, and the only way that gets done is to visit the doctor. There is no substitute (short of telemedicine if that's the only option) for a face-to-face visit with the physician. So why is this still an issue?

Well, men appear to have no shortage of dumb reasons. "I don't want to ask for directions." "I don't want to show that I have no knowledge of a particular topic." These are typical foolish sentiments that Dr. Glenn Good, an expert on masculinity and the psychology of men at the University of Florida, highlighted in a statement to the *Huffington Post.* The American Heart Association expanded on this issue, exploring other bird-brained but genuine excuses for not taking proper medical care of oneself. These include:

- "I don't have a doctor."
- "I don't have insurance."
- "I don't have time."
- "I don't want to spend the money."
- "I'd rather 'tough it out.'"

So here we are in 2020s, and men are still playing the stoic Marlboro Man of decades ago. Along with this macho BS, the lame justifications listed earlier may seem silly and trivial, but they stand up to scrutiny. Indeed, men will say and do just about anything to avoid the doctor's office. What is a spouse, girlfriend, friend, or other loved one to do to combat this foolish and boneheaded behavior? I have a few suggestions:

Show him this section of the book and read to him how lives have been saved and countless suffering (physical, emotional, *and* financial) has been averted by a simple visit to the doctor.

Get on the web and research "Why Men Avoid the Doctor" and show your XY chromosomal friend the potential disasters in not going.

Play on his conscience. If he won't do it for himself, at least he can do it for his life-partner, his children, his friends, coworkers, and community.

Read to him that hypertension, diabetes, prostate cancer, colon cancer, and cardiovascular diseases are relatively common in Western-society men and that these conditions can often be cured or effectively treated if recognized early.

"Scare him straight." Tell him about someone you know who avoided the doctor only to learn that a condition has gone too far, or worse yet, caused an unexpected death to occur in a guy who appeared to be "healthy as a horse."

Most men, when pushed, will listen to reason. But there will still be some guys out there who, despite your best efforts, will resist. At that point, radical measures may be needed. You might have your doctor call him (if the doctor is willing) to stress the importance of a physical. You might have a friend (preferably male), clergy member, trusted relative, or grown child work him over as well. You can also play the "Don't you want to dance at 'fill in the blank's' wedding?" (Insert child or grandchild's name there.)

It's going to take a cultural shift for men to man-up and take control of their health. I fear it is an uphill battle, but one well worth fighting. Men: It's time to drop the macho act and drop your pants for the doctor. It's the right thing to do.

Avoidant attitudes are not the only attitudes that need readjusting. Perhaps just as bad as men neglecting their health is the ongoing stigmatization of mental illness.

Let's End the Stigma of Mental Illness

Sadly, mental illness is still stigmatized in the United States and all over the globe. In the public arena, we widely speak of confronting racism and sexism and advocate for diversity and respect among certain designated groups, but the perceptions and attitudes toward people who suffer emotional illness continue to be negative and misguided.

According to mentalhealthfirstaid.org, some disturbing statistics are revealing:

- Nearly half of adult Americans will experience mental health or substance abuse challenges.
- Five percent of people 18 or older will experience mental illness in any given year.
- In adults in any given year, 14.4% have one, 5.8% have two, and 6% have three or more mental illness issues.
- Half of all mental illness begins by age 14, and three-quarters by age 24.

For further enlightening numbers, you can visit the website of the National Alliance on Mental Health.

Mental disorders come with many diagnoses. The major ones are anxiety, bipolar, schizophrenia, Asperger's, autism spectrum, psychosis, major depressive disorder, panic attacks, antisocial personality disorder, and social anxiety disorders. These and others are described in the *DSM-5*, the diagnostic and statistical manual used by psychiatrists to codify mental disease.

It used to be thought that mental illness, or "madness" as it was called years ago, was a moral or personal shortcoming. Advances in medical science, especially in brain imaging, psychobiology, and neuroscience, lead to the conclusion that mental illness is most surely none other than a medical disease, really no different than any other disease. The altered and dysfunctional actions of neurotransmitters and other chemicals in the brain and central nervous system are what is really behind mental illness, not moral or personal faults.

And yet, people who suffer from these problems are still seen as somehow deficient or lacking in either character, moral fiber, or both. It is time that this attitude ceases.

Advances in treatment aimed at restoring some or most of the neurochemical balance to a person's brain chemistry has vastly improved patient outcomes and prognoses. But even among insurance companies, health plans, and in the legal and political forums, mental illness and its sufferers are still the subject of prejudice and even scorn. This has to stop. And the only ways it can stop is by educating everyone about the medical facts and basis for mental illness and to keep talking about and fine-tuning policy, medical therapy, and the law.

All of us are somehow touched by mental illness. I can think of no one who does not personally, or through a family member or friend, know someone affected by the challenges and pain of mental illness. It is truly the one health issue that everyone should be carefully considering.

The laws about who and under what circumstances treatment must be instituted to protect an unstable mentally ill person from himself or others varies widely. Some of the laws, I've learned from friends and patients, can be very unfair to the families of the mentally ill person. Personal freedom is often protected more than enforcing needed therapy on a truly dangerous mentally ill person. I've seen this time and again.

I understand that personal freedom is an inherently primary right. But when a mentally ill person is shown repeatedly to be a threat, many states make it difficult, past the immediate crisis, to enforce continuing therapy. I know this for a fact because I've seen it firsthand. The issue of enforcing much-needed therapy upon people who are a danger to themselves or others is a contentious one, I'll admit. So is the issue of how insurance and disability carriers will handle claims and reimbursement for the mentally ill. But I've no doubt that there needs to be change—personal, legal, and social—to see mental illness clearly for what it is: a medical disease, first and foremost.

While we are on the topic of mental illness, the upsetting rise in the number of suicides in the United States is worth discussing. There are reasons behind that trend that might surprise you.

Why the Increase in Suicide?

With the recent apparent suicides of two very high-profile people, the public's attention has shifted to this most serious and morose subject. Designer Kate Spade and chef/media star Anthony Bourdain had everything to live for, on the surface: wealth, power, fame, and the privilege that all of that buys. But because no one is immune to illness, and depression is certainly a medical illness, it comes as no surprise that these two famous people suffered the same fate as luminaries such as Marilyn Monroe, Ernest Hemingway, and photographer Diane Arbus.

Time Magazine covered this issue a few years ago and quoted some grim stats:

- There has been a 28% increase in suicide rates from 1999 to 2016.
- Almost 45,000 people killed themselves in our country in 2016.
- There has been a 70% increase in suicide rates among girls from 2010 to 2016.

Having known people who have suffered from depression and anxiety much of my life, I can understand firsthand the pain and struggle people go through. Those not afflicted cannot truly grasp what it means to be so anxious and depressed as to reach the point where Spade and Bourdain got.

But why the increase? Theories abound.

First, understand that depression, anxiety, and the ultimate demon, suicide, have a neurochemical basis. Without getting too technical, our brains—all of our brains—are changing, and not for the better. Our chemicals that regulate mood and outlook—including serotonin, dopamine, norepinephrine, and others—are being messed with by our lifestyles. FOMO, or "fear of missing out," is likely a culprit. People on social media are being fed a constant barrage of what life, in their minds, "should be" like, and anything that falls short means failure.

Also, the rise of obesity and its harpy-like sisters of cardiovascular disease, joint disease, and diabetes, compel us to take more meds, and many of these medications, as reported in today's multiple media outlets, can actually *cause* depression.

Add in the dire situation of the world, with the pollution-related assault on our planet, our lives under consistent threat (with the threat of weapons of mass destruction in these contentious political times), the toxic social environment of racism and injustice and guns killing our children, and certainly the COVID-19 pandemic of recent days, it is small wonder people are depressed.

What to do? Well, if someone talks or threatens suicide, always take it seriously. Also, keep the National Suicide Prevention Lifeline in mind: 1-800-273-8255. Encourage de-stigmatization of mental illness. Get help, in whatever way you can: psychiatrists, psychotherapists, social workers, and related professionals are vital.

Medication can help, but it is not the only or necessarily the best answer. A change in lifestyle is! Eat better. Exercise. Get sunshine.

Get out of bad relationships. Have faith. Pray. Don't live beyond your means. Keep your friends close. And look up cognitive behavioral therapy. Practice it. It's not easy, but it works.

Suicide can be defeated. I know; trust me.

When mental illness—particularly anxiety, depression, and the possibility of suicide—become a problem big enough to merit professional help, therapy and medication can help. One therapeutic breakthrough has received a great deal of attention. You may have heard about it. It's based on an injectable anesthetic that has been used since the 1950s in human and veterinary medicine. Called ketamine, it's a drug, like its evil cousin fentanyl, that has been used on the street by drug abusers. It's too bad these two valuable and essential pharmaceuticals have gotten such a bad name (like the "Michael Jackson drug," propofol), because we in medicine who know what we are doing, use them to greatly benefit patients.

Is Ketamine the New Magic Bullet Against Depression?

In my career as an anesthesiologist, I've used ketamine thousands of times as an adjunct in my anesthesia regimen. This drug was developed decades ago and has been used by anesthesia and veterinary practitioners to place humans and animals in a "dissociative state," a frame of consciousness that straddles the borders of sedation, pain relief, and a blissful "I don't care" attitude.

It has been found that this agent, when administered intravenously or by nasal aerosol, has been remarkably effective at reducing deep depression and anxiety in a rapid fashion.

This has been described as perhaps the most exciting development in psychopharmacology in years. Drugs that normally took weeks or even months to effect a positive change in mood and emotional outlook now appear to have taken a back seat to ketamine.

The use of ketamine in clinical psychiatry has even been purported to rapidly reverse suicidal behavior in some patients who have not responded to other medications.

Ketamine, which is neither narcotic like morphine nor sedative like Valium, is truly in a class by itself. It can be given intramuscularly, intravenously, and by nasal spray. The newer uses for it, to treat anxiety and depression, are given intravenously and by nasal spray. It has been found that a dose of 0.5 mg per kg of body weight given nasally can have a profound and rapid effect on improving mood and reducing anxiety.

One drawback, however, is that the effects may be short-lived—days or weeks—unlike traditional SSRI, SNRI, and other medications that reach a steady state in the body and last for as long as the drug is taken. Also, ketamine therapy may need to be repeated at regular, more frequent intervals.

Side effects can include fast heartbeat, a rise in blood pressure, vivid dreams, excessive salivation, and dysphoria, which is usually short-lived.

Certainly, from the studies being conducted, ketamine therapy is showing promise in psychiatric care that has been wanting due to the lack of effective, rapid, and profound therapy. My best advice to those considering ketamine therapy is to consider the following:

- Repeated dosing may be needed.
- It's best to find a study or center using this therapy that is affiliated with a teaching hospital or medical school.
- Its use should be reserved for rapid relief of moderate-to-severe depression and anxiety, or disorders resistant to other therapies.
- Any clinic involved in this therapy should have accreditation, adequately trained staff (anesthesia personnel are ideal), and safety measures to monitor the patient.

- It can be a "quick fix," but the underlying condition still needs ongoing treatment.

So, yes, ketamine may be the rapid, short-term answer that psychiatry has been looking for to help moderate-to-severe and/or treatment-resistant depression and anxiety. But more studies need to be done. Let's hope this weapon in the fight for better mental health becomes better understood and fine-tuned to a higher degree of effective application.

Perhaps even more impressive as an oft-hoped-for answer to a thorny clinical problem is the tremendous strides recently made in treating a devil of a disease: sickle cell. Although the "cure" appears too expensive and the therapy too labor intensive for wide application right now, the hope is that this type of technology will be more extensively applied to sickle cell sufferers and to others with treatment-amenable genetically related diseases.

Do You Believe in Miracles?
The NIH Has Achieved One

Recently on *60 Minutes*, the CBS Sunday night television magazine, the story of a young woman from Florida who suffered (yes, as in past tense) from sickle cell disease discussed her virtual cure from the condition using gene therapy. The nation, and 8.4 million viewers, were astounded and moved. So was I.

I have a very personal connection to where this treatment for sickle cell disease, and potentially many others, was developed: the National Institutes of Health, or NIH. In the summer of 1953, my late father came to the NIH to do his endocrine fellowship at the fledgling institute, which is now arguably the premiere medical research institute in the world. I often joke with friends that if it wasn't for the NIH and my dad being a physician, I would have never had the good fortune to grow up in a community like Bethesda.

Fast forward to the summer of 2019, where I was helping my friend with his treatments for autoimmune disease at NIH. There, through my friend, I met the man behind the quite miraculous cure (!) of the Florida woman's sickle cell: John Tisdale, MD. I spoke briefly with Dr. Tisdale, an affable man and obviously brilliant researcher, who was helpful in treating my friend's wife for her lymphoma years before. (That's another miracle story.)

In the *60 Minutes* segment, Dr. John LaPook featured Dr. Tisdale and the novel and groundbreaking approach to genetic therapy he employed to treat patients with sickle cell. LaPook also interviewed the director of the NIH, Dr. Francis Collins, who almost committed to using the "C" word (cure) in discussing genetic therapy for sickle cell. The discussions with them, along with the compelling and inspiring interview of the patient in question, made for great drama. I can't think of anyone who was not moved by the story.

Essentially, the science behind the genetic therapy is this: Stem cells are removed from the patient and then the patient is treated with chemotherapy to destroy any remaining stem cells in the body. Afterward, "correct" DNA is substituted for the faulty section of DNA that codes for expression of a disease—in this case, sickle cell. Then in an astounding twist, deactivated (non-disease-causing) HIV, the virus that leads to AIDS in many patients, is used to carry the corrected DNA material to the cells of the patient's body by infusing (injecting) the new material into the patient. It appears that the very thing that makes HIV so dangerous—its ability to transfer DNA into cells all over the human body—is the very thing that makes it, when deactivated as a disease carrier, a great deliverer of healing DNA.

So why should you care about this? This is why: Other than the great news for sickle cell sufferers and their loved ones, Dr. Collins has proposed that because the DNA defects of 7,000 diseases have been mapped out to date, the potential to use the same or similar technology to "cure" other diseases may already be out there. Think what that means for the future and for patients with cancer, neurologic, endocrine, autoimmune, and a host of other horrible and formerly "hopeless" diseases! If it worked for the previously uncurable sickle cell disease, why not for others?

So take heart. There may be a miracle just around the corner for you, a family member, or friend. If you are told that what you have is not treatable, it is certainly encouraging to know that medical science just might have something in the wings for you. And while other treatments may buy you time (see the recent reports in the reduction of cancer deaths, particularly melanoma), researchers are likely busy addressing the very conditions from which you suffer.

The sickle cell "cure" story is a compelling one, as is an established and more widespread therapeutic intervention: bone marrow transplantation. That technology, which has saved untold lives over the years, has also made headlines recently, but in a tragic way.

Is Bone Marrow Donation Safe?

A heroic but tragic case of altruism turned deadly recently as a high school principal in New Jersey lost his life donating bone marrow to help a stranger in France. Derrick Nelson, a high school principal and a man with a history of sleep apnea and sickle cell anemia carrier state, underwent harvesting of bone marrow under local anesthesia to help someone on the other side of the world. After the procedure, he was unable to speak and eventually lapsed into a coma. He ultimately died weeks later.

The press has no reports I am aware of that reveal the cause of his death. But I have my theories.

First, understand that death from bone marrow donation is exceedingly rare, but not unheard of. Complications can include infection, bleeding, and in the most severe circumstances, embolization. Emboli are small particles or tissue entities—like fat, blood clots, or even trapped gases like air—that can enter blood vessels and travel via the circulatory system to the heart, lungs, and even the brain and other vital organs. Emboli due to blood elements often come in the form of clots and are, perhaps, the most common and well-known. Deep vein thrombosis, often in the leg, can cause a clot to dislodge from the wall of a vein and travel to the heart and lungs, causing a serious pulmonary embolus. Amniotic fluid embolization during childbirth can similarly cause a serious clinical picture when amniotic tissue traverses from the uterus into the general circulation. Fat emboli can enter the circulation during orthopedic surgery and after injury to large bones of the body, such as the femur. Also, some people have a genetic or acquired propensity to develop blood clots, requiring them to be anticoagulated (blood-thinned) in order to prevent serious complications from clots.

In the case of Mr. Nelson, he unfortunately had a number of medical issues that might have contributed to his death. His sleep apnea did put him at risk for anesthesia, even though it was done under local with sedation and not under riskier general anesthesia. Also, he appeared to be overweight, which always places people at extra risk for anesthesia, as is the case with a person with sickle cell disease (although it is unclear whether he suffered any clinical manifestations of this disease). My pet theory, due to the clinical picture, is that he might have suffered an embolization of bone marrow fat or other cellular material during or shortly after the procedure, although I cannot say for sure.

What happened to this poor man, who heroically lost his life in service to others, serves as a rare but sad lesson. Although bone marrow donation is extremely safe, there are risks involved, just as there are risks in any medical intervention. The risks can be quite small, but other health factors, like extra pounds, sleep apnea, sickle cell disease of unknown severity, or risks that are unknown at the time of the procedure can contribute to complications. This is in no way a discouragement to bone marrow donation or any other medical procedure. It is, however, a warning to gather as much information as you can about your own health before medical interventions of any kind to help the people taking care of you do the safest job possible. And whenever it is feasible, you can do things to protect yourself, like lose weight, get your sleep apnea under control, and do other smart things like quitting smoking, managing your health problems through better habits, and taking your medication as prescribed to help mitigate risks. Although this case is a tragic example of the adage "no good deed ever goes unpunished," it should not deter anyone from doing the right thing.

The sad and untimely death of Mr. Nelson in the preceding section brings me to a related topic: How we as a society approach terminal illness. So much of our healthcare dollars are spent in the last six months of life and I'm not sure this is sustainable. Is it time we rethink our own mortality?

Bone marrow donation is generally safe, when done skillfully and with the right preprocedure preparation and evaluation. It is an extreme measure used to help the ill recover and has saved many lives. The donors do take risks, as you can see, when they give this essential tissue to others.

Incredibly, one increasingly common and risky practice that people appear happy to take on is vaping, a habit that a growing number of studies is proving to be rather unsafe.

The Truth About Vaping:
What E-Cig Makers Don't Want You to Know

As a reader of my hometown newspaper, the *Washington Post*, I am taken aback by the frequent full-page ads for Juul, the vaping product that touts itself as a better alternative to tobacco smoking. These ads leave me skeptical and even a bit nauseous. The *Post*'s ads often show a smiling former smoker and includes a quote from that person as to why he or she took up vaping. I, for one, am not convinced of the alleged benefits.

A recent report by Michael Blaha, MD, MPH, and director of clinical research at the Johns Hopkins Ciccarone Center for the Prevention of Heart Disease, clearly and convincingly summarized the falsehoods inherent in the pro-vaping arguments, writing of the myths regarding the supposed benefits of vaping. He debunks all of them. They include:

- Vaping, although not true smoking, is the inhalation of nicotine. Tobacco contains about 7,000 chemicals, most of which are toxic. While vaping may expose you to less chemicals, the addictive and toxic effects of nicotine, which include a rise in pulse, blood pressure, and adrenaline, are still there and are even magnified.
- People who vape are frequently still smokers. The makers of vaping products say it is a better alternative to smoking, but the truth lies elsewhere. Studies have shown that most people who vape also continue to abuse cigarettes.
- Vaping is attracting a younger and more vulnerable crowd, especially in its flavored varieties of vaping products. This hooks younger people on a product proven to be harmful to the cardiovascular system (at a minimum) and other body systems (central nervous system, respiratory system) as well.

- As mentioned before, nicotine, when concentrated in vapor, causes a spike in blood pressure and heart rate, and can cause undue cardiac stimulation and unwanted cardiovascular effects in vulnerable people (i.e., patients with existing high blood pressure, heart disease, and heart rhythm problems). Nicotine is not benign and should not be marketed as such. There have been reports that vaping may expose the user to lead and heavy metals, which are proven toxins.

The journal *Physician's Weekly* has also weighed in. It recently cited some confirmatory evidence, as well as additional damning info:

Only 10% of nearly 1,300 smokers in one study were able to quit smoking cigarettes by vaping. Vaping has been shown to have deleterious effects, due to high nicotine exposure, on developing teenage brains. They quote a study in an American Heart Association journal that reveals the flavorings in vaping products may damage blood vessels and even the reproductive tract. Nicotine in e-cigarettes impaired beneficial acetylcholine-mediated blood vessel dilation, causing arterial stiffness and a rise in blood pressure and heart rate. Even protective cough reflexes were reduced in another study, and still another showed inflammatory effects on the lungs and deleterious changes in the cells of the lungs that help prevent infection.

With vaping rates having increased among teens an impressive 900% from 2011 to 2015, it's easy to see why health advocacy groups have gotten fired up about the lies that vaping is a safe alternative to smoking. Clearly, both are bad for you. And it's time that the FDA, the public, and the press cut through the haze of obfuscations and hyped claims and call out vaping for what it is: another way to poison oneself through the inhalation of toxins that damage the lungs and the cardiovascular, nervous, immune, and reproductive systems.

So stop rationalizing, and just quit it. If you need help, there are great resources on offer at SmokeFree.gov. I urge you to check it out.

What Do You Do When Life Isn't Worth Living?

Let me tell you a true story. A person I know, who is 89 and has a number of significant chronic diseases (none of them "terminal"), has been admitted to the hospital each month for the past nine months. Her stays in the hospital vary from overnight to a few days, and are mostly for dehydration, infections of the lungs or urinary tract, intractable constipation, and uncontrolled blood pressure. She is on a total of 15 medications, cannot leave her home, and is in chronic pain. Her days at home are spent in bed, sometimes watching TV, reading, or doing crossword puzzles.

Now, when I read a recent article by Paula Span in the *New York Times* about a surgeon in Denver who does not operate on patients who are overly frail and elderly, it really hit home. In fact, it jogged my memory about a surgical case I was involved with two decades ago. A 90-year-old nursing home patient, who was bedridden, fell out of bed and broke his hip. He came to the operating room for a "hip pinning," where the broken bones are put roughly back in place. He was all twisted up like a pretzel, moaning in pain, and could not speak intelligibly. The poor man was in agony. I kept asking myself "Why are we doing this case?" As I was giving the spinal anesthetic, I wondered whether we physicians were really doing this unfortunate human being a disservice by prolonging a life that, for all appearances, was rife with pain and suffering. It was hard for me to imagine this man, who had lived a full life, looking forward to anything. I knew perfectly well that this was not my call to make— that I should never "play God"—but I pondered over the poor man's plight (and our actions) nonetheless.

The article is a challenge to the belief that we must, as a society, generally treat patients medically and surgically at all costs, despite how old, ill, or poor their quality of life. Certainly, there are exceptions to this tenet, but for the most part, Americans believe that our far-advanced medical care, with its life-prolonging and lifesaving qualities, is to be wielded whenever and wherever an insistent family member or loved one dictates. Indeed, family members often clash when an elderly parent is chronically and seriously ill, only to be saved by heroic, advanced medical care. Further complicating the issue is money. The cost of continuing care, as well as the substantial estates that many elderly possess, are two major issues that divide families near the end of a parent's or other relative's life.

Many questions emerge here. One is, where have we come in terms of life span? You'd be shocked to learn. In 1900, the average white man lived, on average, 47 years, a white woman, 49. The numbers for blacks were worse: 33 for men and 34 for women. By 1960, the numbers across the board had improved to 67 for white men, 74 for white women, and 61 and 66 for black men and women, respectively. Today, the averages are up by a decade to a decade and change. Clearly, the things that killed people at a younger age in 1900 and 1960, like infectious disease, cancer, cardiovascular disease, and childbirth, are being medically mitigated and in some cases vanquished.

Another question concerns quality of life. We all know what that is: the ability to enjoy, participate in, look forward to, or otherwise value existence, both in health and during chronic illness. Certainly, medical and surgical care in our country has enabled this to occur. Medications, surgical techniques, and other groundbreaking therapies (stem cells, radiation, gene therapy, etc.) have enabled many to live longer and, in some cases, better lives. I say "some cases," because of the example I used to begin my article: a person, pushing 90, on a number of expensive and side-effect-inducing medications, who is in and out of the hospital and is really just clinging to life. I have no doubt the person in question would flunk the Denver surgeon's frailty test mentioned in the *New York Times* article.

Where does this sentiment (i.e., the justification of the restriction of some forms of medical and surgical care) leave us as a society? The question is complicated and will only get more complicated. In previous chapters, I have written about the importance of lifestyle changes, the contribution of obesity to poor health, the ever-growing number of medications and supplements patients take, the rising colorectal cancer rates in younger people, and the alarming increase in opioid dependence and overdose deaths. These factors, among others, are the recipe for the following scenario: a culture where people are on more medication, with more frail elderly and people living extended, but not necessarily better, lives. I have no doubt life span will continue to rise. I also have no doubt that these longer lives will be burdened by chronic disease. I base this conclusion on the shocking statistic that nearly 70% of Americans are overweight or obese, with that trend not ending anytime soon. In a prior chapter, I called this problem "the mother of all diseases." I still contend that this alone will lead to an economic stress severe enough to compel the forces that dictate the cost, allocation, and availability of healthcare in the United States to make these hard choices about who will get treatment for certain diseases and who will not.

Simply put, the status quo is not sustainable. As I've said many times, we do not merely have a "healthcare crisis" in our country. We, more importantly, have a "health crisis." But no one seems to want to talk about that. Until we do discuss this, openly and frankly, and implement some of the measures I alluded to about the obesity problem and substance abuse, the decision over whether to treat the too frail or too chronically sick will answer itself. After all, money still talks and makes the world go round—the economic factor, not medical ethics, not the judicial system, will be *the* deciding factor regarding this thorny issue.

As the preceding example illustrates, things can get contentious when a family member or loved one is dying. All kinds of issues emerge and difficult conversations are likely to arise. Is there a better way to deal with that when the situation inevitably arises? There is.

How to Avoid Family Conflicts
When a Parent Is Ill or Dying

It's going to happen to almost everyone: conflicts with family in dealing with a sick and ailing parent. The parent's illness itself may cause disagreement and strife, but this issue is best handled well before illness and disability occurs—through thoughtful discussion and careful planning. But there are other factors, dealing more with the children themselves, that complicate matters.

A family I know had vast income discrepancies among the children. The eldest, who asserted herself and coerced the ailing mother into giving her power of attorney and making her executor, got the mother to agree to give her an extra $50,000 payout at the time of the parent's death. This obviously did not sit well with the other children. Because she had made less money than the other offspring, she thought she was somehow justified in this. The siblings disagreed, and things were unpleasant for a long time thereafter.

Another situation involved a family where the three daughters were in different places in their lives. One had severe obsessive-compulsive disorder (OCD) and needed help herself. Another was a jet-setting Wall Street–type who lived in another country and had little to do with the family. The third child lived locally with their mother and was compelled to do much of the coordinating of her mother's care and finances. Clearly, conflicts arose regarding the role each child should or could play regarding care of the ailing mother.

These are typical examples of what can happen when rivalries, unresolved grievances, and income disparities reemerge when parents get sick.

As Belinda Hulin wrote recently on Care.com, there are three main factors that cause problems when a parent is failing: roles and rivalries, sharing responsibilities, and spending and needs assessments. How families deal with these issues will dictate how smoothly things will go when a parent is sick and dying.

When there is more than one child in a family, there will be more than one opinion on decisions as diverse as doctor and hospital choice, hospice or no hospice, advanced directives, power of attorney, finances, and funeral arrangements. Old rivalries are likely to emerge, and power struggles between children, as well as between children and their parents, will emerge. These struggles, of course, only add to the stress of dealing with the illness at hand.

Oftentimes, one child will live closer to the ailing parent than the other(s) and this will often dictate who becomes the care coordinator or even primary caretaker. Resentment over this issue can be intense and lead to further conflict and argument between the offspring.

Children often have vastly differing financial situations, and this often results in disagreement over how much money is spent—and how it is spent—for the care of the sick parent. Many children today are poised to inherit considerable funds, and this possibility results, many times, in bitter disputes over spending.

What to do? There are no easy answers. One approach is to have children and their parents sit down and hash out these issues long before the need arises. Although uncomfortable and difficult to do, this approach can save a lot of headache and heartache down the line. Enlisting the help of an eldercare attorney and the family's financial advisor can also be beneficial. Even clergy can play a role.

But communication is vital. Honest and open discussion between parents and all their children as to living wills, power of attorney, advanced directives, financial constraints and limitations, choices as to who will deliver healthcare and where, and perhaps most important, the role each child will play in the process, will go a long way in making a difficult situation a bit easier.

Don't wait until an elder parent is ill. The time to talk is now.

In the earlier personal example, I said the 89-year-old person in question was on 15 prescription medications. That's clearly an outlier, but it is not unprecedented. That brings me to my next topic: the coming medication shortages.

Generic Drugs: Shortages, Price Gouging, and Other Crimes

Much attention has been paid in recent years to the unfortunate reality of drug shortages and wild price inflation in the United States. The reasons for this serious problem are complex, but the bottom line is (as always in these types of things) money. Almost everyone who has had a need for chronic or even short-term drug therapy has experienced the frustration and upset of having to pay unreasonably high prices for prescribed treatment. Many of these same patients have been told that there is a shortage of medications that have been in existence for decades.

Before I can speak about what you can do to help yourself when drugs are too costly or unavailable, I'll explain how this dilemma came about.

First, it is important to realize that prescription drugs are either available as brand name or generics. Over 85% of the prescriptions written in our country are for the generic, or "off-patent," version of a medication. Because the majority of prescribed medications are generic, many of these agents have been on the market for decades.

One would think that because these medicines have been used for so long, and their safety and effectiveness have stood the test of time, they would be the least costly. In many cases, that is true. But in some critical areas of treatment, such as in cancer care, antibiotic therapy, anesthetics, and even something as simple as intravenous salt solutions, forces have conspired to create shortages that have led to price gouging by certain large generic suppliers.

In 2007, the FDA said that 154 drugs had become scarce or were no longer on the market. By 2012, that number had grown to more than 300. What is causing this? Recently, a report in the journal *Global IT* quoted the National Center for Biotechnology Information, saying the following:

- Manufacturing difficulties caused a decrease in the production of updated drugs.
- Shortages of raw materials caused delays in crucial materials.
- Natural disasters caused shortages in inventories.
- FDA regulatory issues tied up production and distribution.
- Simple supply-and-demand issues disrupted the stock of necessary medication.

But there are other, more sinister reasons behind the alarming shortages and increase in prices that have resulted in staggering increases in medicines for gout (colchicine, up 50-fold), heart failure (digoxin, up 6-fold), and arrhythmias (isoproterenol, up 5-fold) over the last five decades. One 62-year-old treatment for the parasitic disease toxoplasmosis is up over 5,000%, from $13 to $750 per tablet! This price increase occurred in 2015 alone, when the company (Turing Pharmaceuticals) acquired rights to the drug.

Health Affairs blog has recently reported that it is the sharp rise in generic drug prices that has affected consumers the most. In February 2016, that journal stated:

> Stronger generic manufacturers ... absorbed numerous
> competitors. ... For many drugs ... a combination of
> supply-chain disruptions, manufacturing problems, FDA
> compliance problems, and business failures ... reduced the
> number of suppliers. As a result ... generic products were
> left with only 2 or 3 active suppliers ... creating a natural
> monopoly. ... While generic drugs are still ... less costly
> than brand-name ... in 2013, one-third of generic drugs
> had a price increase, with about 10% of generics posting an
> increase of 50% or more.

The article goes on to say that this caused "President Obama to issue an Executive Order ... directing the FDA to take steps to alleviate 'a serious and growing threat to public health.'"

So what is the patient to do about the fact that, according to the U.S. Department of Health and Human Services, 22% of the top generics reviewed in the decade prior to 2014 rose in price faster than inflation? How can we all get a handle on this ever-growing concern?

I have a few ideas:

- Always ask your doctor for the least-expensive alternative for your medication. If he or she does not know the answer, check with your insurance plan to see which blood pressure, blood thinner, or diabetic medication is most cost-effective and meets with your doctor's approval for your treatment plan.
- Better yet, take better care of yourself by embracing better habits. Restrict saturated fat, sugar, and refined carbohydrates from your diet. Exercise. Lose weight. Stop smoking. Think of the freedom you'll have (as well as the extra money) by not having to take as many medications.
- Always ask your doctor if you need to be on medications that a former practitioner had put you on. Oftentimes, conditions

improve or resolve themselves altogether, yet patients are still on medications for conditions that are no longer problems. Americans are overmedicated. I can't stress this enough.

- Get politically active. I know it seems like an impossible task, but if enough citizens complained to their senators and congresspersons about the predatory monopolies in the drug industry, some improvements might be made.
- Shop for health plans that are large enough and strong enough to have negotiated better pricing for necessary medication.
- Consider acupuncture, yoga, meditation, herbal, psycho- or physiotherapy, or other nondrug modalities for some of your medical issues. They are almost always better for you than pills.

While we are on the topic of drug shortages, it's instructive to note the impact drug scarcity has had during the recent COVID-19 pandemic with regard to the possible need for artificial ventilation. Most laymen misunderstand what "being on a ventilator" entails. Here's what you should know and the questions you should ask if this unlikely scenario arises for you or a loved one.

What If I Need a Ventilator?

Among the many fears people have expressed during the COVID-19 epidemic in our country, one question appears uppermost in Americans' minds: "What if I need a ventilator?"

I hope to clarify what assisted ventilation from a ventilator (or respirator) entails and give tips for you and your family or patient advocate should that unlikely but daunting prospect arise.

Much has been said in the press, on the street, and among our government leaders about the potential shortage of ventilators during the present COVID-19 outbreak. Many people misunderstand what it means to be ventilated or "on" a ventilator. As an anesthesiologist for nearly three and a half decades who has managed artificially ventilated patients in operating rooms, ICUs, and other clinical settings, I feel it is important you understand the concept and mechanical details of artificial ventilation.

When a patient is rendered anesthesia-induced unconscious for surgery or is in the ICU and intubated for treatment of respiratory failure, the need for artificial ventilation arises. Since 1870, when Dr. Trendelenburg performed the first intubation in Germany, I and specially trained doctors, nurses, and assistants like me have intubated people so they may be mechanically ventilated.

Intubation is the act of placing a breathing tube into a patient's trachea (windpipe) so that mechanical ventilation can be achieved. The breathing tube is generally placed either through the patient's mouth or nostril. More rarely, it is done surgically via a tracheostomy through the patient's anterior (front) neck. This is achieved with a tool called a laryngoscope or with the use of a fiberoptic scope.

This "breathing for" the patient is, by definition, the forced inspiration of oxygen-enriched gas and the exhalation of carbon dioxide–rich gas. Sometimes we anesthesiologists or critical care doctors "paralyze" patients with neuromuscular blocking drugs (paralytics) to ease our ability to ventilate for them. Other times, patients are not paralyzed and allowed some degree of autorespiration, usually with support from the ventilatory apparatus. In almost all cases, patients are sedated, especially in the ICU setting, in order to permit tolerating the physical, mental, and emotional trauma of intubation and ventilation.

A lot has been written recently about the potential shortage of ventilators needed to deal with the present crisis. I will not debate here whether that concern is legitimate or not. But we certainly have come a long way in that, during the polio epidemic of the 1950s, the shortfall of "iron lung" ventilation systems was made up for by other means, namely the squeezing of a bag (like a bellows) by a team of medical students pressed into service to offer temporary round-the-clock ventilatory support.

Already in this nation, elective surgeries are being canceled to divert anesthesia machine ventilators for possible use in the novel coronavirus outbreak. Also, automobile manufacturers are being asked, as other industries are, to quickly retool their plants to churn out more ventilators. Whether that will be sufficient to meet the potential need for intubated patients in respiratory failure is not yet clear.

But what is clear is this: Being intubated is physically, emotionally, and mentally taxing. People have a right to be concerned. But do realize that only the sickest minority of COVID-19 patients will *require* intubation and ventilation. The odds are in your favor, depending on your age and preexisting medical state, that this will never come to pass for you.

Should the situation arise, it is important to ask the providers if there are sufficient sedatives and sleep drugs (like benzodiazepines and propofol), painkillers (narcotics like morphine and fentanyl), and paralytics (like pancuronium, rocuronium, and vecuronium) available to keep you comfortable and immobile to achieve effective ventilation. I know these are difficult questions, but they are, in these times of drug shortages, legitimate.

I truly hope you never need to ask them.

Drugs, ventilators, intravenous fluids, viral testing kits—the potential short supply of all these vital medical cogs have received much attention. But what about personnel?

Drugs Are Not the Only Thing That Will Be in Short Supply

Recently, I have had the opportunity to guide three close friends through the intricacies of the American healthcare system. Other than some apparent substandard care in all three cases (conditions and illnesses not addressed, misdiagnoses, and inattentive staff) one factor appeared common to all of my friends: shortages.

Whether it was from a doctor or nursing shortage, a lack of hospital beds or a shortage of medication and intravenous fluid supplies, I found it surprising that the allegedly "best" medical care in the world should suffer from such shortcomings. But on reflection, I can see why. I've addressed drug shortages before, so let's talk about shortages of skilled providers.

First, the doctors. It is apparent that the number of doctors available to treat patients is falling, and this will likely only get worse. According to data from the American Association of Medical Colleges (AAMC), "if all Americans had utilization patterns similar to non-Hispanic white populations with insurance in metropolitan areas, the U.S. would need an additional 95,100 doctors immediately." The same AAMC report projects that by 2030 (less than a decade away), the doctor shortage is estimated to be as high as 121,300. In the next 10 years, the U.S. population is expected to increase by 11%, and the number of Americans over age 65 years will grow by 50%. Because older people account for the most medical care, this surely will be a problem.

So too with nursing staff. Recently, a survey of chief nursing officers showed that 72% surveyed said that they've been affected by at least "moderate" nursing shortages, and 40% have said that shortages were having a "considerable" or "great" impact on patient satisfaction.

As well, there is a phenomenon in hospitals called emergency department diversion, where that department essentially has to operate as a hospital ward, sometimes for days at a time, for lack of available regular hospital beds. My friend here in Washington, D.C., had to transfer his care to the NIH from a university hospital because the latter wanted to treat him for two days or more in the emergency department.

All three of my friends recently seeking care have experienced at least one and sometimes two of the previously mentioned challenges. Combine that with potential future drug and other essential therapy supply shortages and it is easy to see why, in the coming years, there will be a real "crisis" in healthcare.

The reasons for shortages are complicated. Certainly, an aging, older, and increasingly chronically sick population is a primary cause. So is an unwillingness of potential medical students to take on the long, hard years of training only to be saddled with enormous debt at the end of their schooling. Also, with over a trillion dollars allocated to healthcare in the federal budget, it is easy to see why the massive expenses required to administer to the health of Americans (who, as I pointed out already, are apparently uneager to take better care of themselves) strain the country's finances. The shortcomings of the system have been nowhere more apparent than in our own Veterans Administration healthcare, where, at least until recently, veterans had to wait months, even years, to get the care they've earned by serving our country.

What's the answer to all this? Sadly, I don't see one. "Medicare for all" surely isn't a solution, because it would probably worsen the doctor shortage and force many hospitals to go out of business unless Medicare reimbursement payment scales are drastically altered. (What young person would go into all that debt to be reimbursed, compared to private insurance, at Medicare's measly rates?) Will people start taking better care of themselves? Knowing human nature and the trends in health, probably not. Perhaps the ever-growing trend in telemedicine will pick up some of the slack, as will possible "breakthrough" therapies.

Until then, be prepared for shortages to continue and perhaps grow, and expect patient care, as well as morbidity and mortality, to worsen.

If up to now you sense that I've painted a dire picture of what healthcare might look like in the coming decades, I'd say you are making a fair assessment. I am a realist, after all, and just report it as I see it. Shortages are real—across the board—as the recent COVID-19 pandemic has illustrated. Testing kits, ventilators, narcotics, sedatives, paralyzing agents for intubation, doctors, nurses, first responders—all these essential elements were or were thought to be in insufficient supply during the recent health disaster.

So what would your average red-blooded American think of doing in this situation? Suing, of course! Getting a lawyer to work his or her magic in the courtroom to financially make up for the real or perceived injustices that were meted out during this time of trouble is always on some patients' minds. It seems to me that the farther I head south on Interstate 95, the more billboards I see for lawyers to "get you the money you deserve" for your terrible outcomes at the hands of quacks and charlatans. Of course, we all know that legal remedies with regard to medical malpractice and malfeasance in normal times, let alone a pandemic, are still viable and reasonable options when things go south medically. Or are they?

Thinking of Suing Your Doctor? Read This First

Many times, in my 40-plus years involved in medicine, I have experienced the nuances and trauma of medical malpractice in all its splendor. I've looked on as medical careers and personal lives were shattered, patients were injured, lawyers rubbed their hands together, and potential codefendants ran for cover. Yes, no word like "malpractice" can quite send a chill up a physician's spine.

But few patients, and perhaps even fewer doctors, really understand what both the definition and process of malpractice is. Simply put, medical malpractice refers to a "tort," a legal term for a civil (as opposed to criminal) wrong, perpetrated by one party on another. It grew out of English Common Law and, despite efforts at reform—including no-fault (as New Zealand has), limited liability (as some states have), and statutes of limitation—medical malpractice is still all too common. It has been estimated that, depending on the specialty, a doctor can expect to be sued every 7 years. Why is this so?

Let's first look at what legally defines medical malpractice. For it to have legally occurred, four criteria must be met. If any one of the four is not met, there are no grounds for a malpractice lawsuit. They are:

1. There must be a doctor–patient relationship.
2. The doctor must have a duty to the patient.
3. The doctor must breach that duty.
4. The breach of the duty must cause harm.

This is where most patients and doctors get tangled up. The reason so many cases never go to trial is that all four of the criteria are often not met. Plaintiff's attorneys should know this; the ones who do know are resistant, rightly so, to take on a case. Sometimes a patient or plaintiff's attorney will go looking for a harm that is supposedly done to a patient, such as lack of consortium (where a patient's relationship with a spouse or partner has allegedly been negatively affected by a physician's action). One case is the patient who had surgery and developed an ugly scar and, as a result, the patient's husband does not want to have sex with the patient. This is an extreme example, but it does occur.

The common reasons patients sue doctors are:

- Lack of informed consent
- Operating on the wrong site
- Delayed or missed diagnosis that eventually caused harm
- Retained surgical instruments in the patient's body
- Adverse drug reactions
- Complications from interventions
- Birth-related injuries, whether immediate or of later onset
- Anesthesia injuries, including brain death, wrongful death, nerve injuries, dental injuries, throat injuries, or eye injuries

And there are plenty more reasons to sue. Lawyers and plaintiffs can harbor vivid imaginations.

There is a standard that physicians are held to in order to determine whether she or he deviated from the standard of care and therefore was negligent in performing medical duties. That standard is usually defined as "what a physician exercising diligence with similar training and experience in the community" would have done in identical or similar circumstances.

Keep in mind that certain jurisdictions, due to demographics, politics, and other factors, can be either more plaintiff- or defendant-friendly. For example, a plaintiff's case tried in Washington, DC, my hometown, is much more likely to go a plaintiff's way, all things being equal, than a case in Arlington, Virginia, a mere two miles from DC. There, defendants fare better.

Also be mindful of the legal arrangements. Most lawyers will only take a case if they see a potential big payout for themselves, as in an injured baby case or a case where a breadwinner for a large family is severely injured. Most plaintiff's attorneys work on a contingency basis, where they get a percentage of the total award. If you consider a lawsuit, you should keep that in mind. Also understand the breakdown of damages. You could be awarded money for additional hospital or medical care, as well as compensatory damages for lost income, future missed earnings, and even putative damages, which punish the defendant for particularly egregious errors or omissions.

But if you do consider suing your doctor, you must recognize all that I've written earlier plus know that:

- The process can be slow—think years.
- Most malpractice cases are settled out of court (i.e., they never go to trial).
- You are unlikely to gain as much financially as you first thought.
- Lawyers may keep a significant portion of the payout.
- Cases can be expensive to prosecute.

I've seen great, dedicated, and skillful doctors get sued, while those who I wouldn't let touch my cat never get sued. Medicine and the law often intersect in capricious ways. Just because a doctor is listed in the NPDB (National Practitioner Data Bank, a repository of malpractice payouts and other disciplinary actions) does not necessarily mean your doctor is not skilled, diligent, or caring. The converse is true as well. Perhaps the best way to protect yourself is to read physicians' reviews online, ask your friends and family, and even visit your state's medical board website to look up your doctor.

But if you feel you must sue, realize this: Most patients seek the courts because they feel the doctor did not care, did not communicate effectively, or when an adverse outcome occurred, did not own up to it and apologize. Studies have shown that doctors who commit these types of errors are more likely to get sued, no matter the outcome of the medical issue, than those who act in an opposite manner.

While we're talking about doctors, it's worthwhile noting another growing trend in American medicine: the role of the D.O. versus the MD.

MD or DO: Does Your Doctor's Degree Matter?

My 1984 Boston University medical school diploma, written in Latin, boldly proclaims me, in large gothic letters, to be a newly minted "Doctoris Medicinae," or "Doctor of Medicine." Long have I stared at those fancy words, identical to the designation used on my late father's medical school diploma from the same institution in 1950.

But what if those letters stood not for doctor of medicine but doctor of osteopathic medicine? Would it matter? Is the training that different? Is my medical skill and knowledge base better or more advanced than that of an osteopathic physician?

The short answer is "no." Osteopathic medical degrees, offered in 35 schools in the United States compared with 141 schools that offer the MD degree, have become widely accepted as equivalent in scope and training when compared to their MD counterparts. Osteopathic medicine grew out of a late-ninteenth-century American tradition in medical practice founded by Andrew Taylor Still. He began a movement of medical education and practice that encompassed training physicians in musculoskeletal manipulation, as well as other more traditional disciplines of established medical knowledge.

Today, the physicians who graduate from these schools, in addition to having received virtually identical training and coursework that is offered at MD-granting schools, also gain additional training (hundreds of hours, depending on the particular D.O. school) of musculoskeletal manipulation as a basis for treating disease. While there is controversy as to the effectiveness of that type of treatment, what is not in question is the D.O.'s acceptance as an equivalent degree to the MD in terms of rights, advanced medical training opportunities (internships, residencies, and fellowships) and licensing, professional associations, and medical leadership roles.

Having said all this, there may be subtle differences in the overall approach to the patient and her/his care. Reflected in that is the tendency for D.O. physicians to concentrate in primary care and internal medicine. This may be due, in part, because osteopathic approach to medicine is viewed by some as more slanted toward treating the whole person than the MD-allopathic model of diagnosis and treatment. One needs look no further than that the D.O.'s training encompasses hands-on manipulation of the human body to understand why this might be the case. While this approach may reflect the tendencies to step outside the allopathic role and move into physical manipulation as an additional approach to heal, there is still controversy, as I have mentioned, about the overall efficacy of this attitude toward healing.

One minor difference to report between D.O. and MD applicants to medical school: The MCAT (Medical College Admission Test) scores and GPAs of D.O. applicants were slightly lower than MD applicants. Whether this is of significance in the overall quality of care delivered by D.O.s is a bit dubious. Still, it is a statistic that has been evaluated. Indeed, I have worked side by side with D.O.s in a variety of clinical settings, both at the general, specialty, and subspecialty level, and have noted no differences in diagnostic skill, quality of care, or any other parameter one might choose to select. But that is anecdotal. The studies on this bear me out, but you are free to search on your own.

So because 20% of all medical school enrollment is now at schools that offer the D.O. degree, you can expect to see a lot more of these professionals treating you in all aspects of medical care in the future. You should also rest assured that these doctors have equivalent training and have passed comparable or identical exams that MDs have completed to practice their arts.

The bottom line here: MD or D.O.? Nowadays, it does not really matter.

Now, a final word about a medical-practice policy that needs attention and changing. Many of you will relate to this.

Medicine's Barbaric Little Secret: IVs Don't Have to Hurt

I was speaking to an old friend, a fellow physician, the other day about what makes hospitalized patients most uncomfortable. Incredibly, one of the things he told me was that when he is doing rounds in the intensive care unit (ICU), the blood drawings for the daily testing take place around 4:00 am. I was shocked! How can patients get adequate rest when someone is jabbing a needle in their arms at that ungodly hour?

This led to a discussion about what doctors and nurses do to patients that border on barbarity. One of them is starting intravenous lines with no local anesthesia on the skin. I consider this one of the medical practice's dirty little secrets. Let me explain.

When I entered anesthesia training in 1986, I was introduced to a practice that has long been the standard of anesthesia personnel, from physician anesthesiologists to nurse anesthetists to anesthesia assistants and pre-op nurses: the use of local anesthesia on the skin to start an IV.

When I was an internal medicine intern and medical student, I witnessed the unnecessary infliction of pain on patients who had their IVs started without local anesthesia, often by inexperienced students and interns. This horrible and immoral practice was considered the norm. It wasn't intentional, it was just the way things were done.

In 1986, as a new anesthesia resident, I was taught how to start an IV and, more important, how to do so relatively painlessly—with the use of less than 1 cc of the local anesthetic lidocaine. What we were taught is still practiced by many in my specialty today. A small wheal (bubble) of local anesthetic is applied with a tiny (and I mean tiny!) needle just where the IV is to be started in the vein. After five seconds, the practitioner can, with virtually *no* pain to the patient, search for and find the proper site for insertion of the IV catheter.

I know this to be true because, in my estimation, I've done this an astounding 80,000 times (you read that right) over a nearly 32-year career.

There is absolutely no reason this should not be standard practice for every patient in need of an IV. The training takes five minutes and the results are dramatic. The amount of lidocaine administered is so minute it causes no ill effects. And the patients are spared the painful ordeal of IV starts, especially when multiple sticks are involved.

My physician friend and I agreed that another area where this can be employed is when an arterial blood gas is drawn. This procedure is even more painful than an IV start. A needle is inserted into an artery to obtain an arterial blood sample for analysis. Let me tell you, it hurts like hell. Yet healthcare personnel still inflict it and patients endure it.

So let this be the year that patients stand up for themselves. Let it be the year that healthcare professionals ease the pain of patients. And let now be the time that I put the message out: This barbaric practice is unnecessary and unwarranted. A touch of lidocaine in the right hands can make all the difference in the world.

CHAPTER 6

Behind the Mask

Who Are Doctors, Really?

Doctors—the people behind the white coats, surgical masks, or at the other end of the endoscopes—are a strange breed of professionals. They study and sacrifice for years to practice the healing arts and sciences, and most of them pay a heavy price in the process. That price is financial, psychological, and physical, and is mitigated with the reasonably realistic promise of a high income at the end of the educational tunnel.

The typical mid-twentieth-century view of a doctor was that of a white male, gentle and reassuring in nature and always quick to reassure and comfort the sick patient and his or her family. Think Marcus Welby, MD, if you are old enough to remember him. In the latter part of the last century, more women and minorities, thankfully, entered medicine to make the healing workforce more diverse. Today, more women and people of color practice medicine in the United States than at any other time since records on this have been kept. And with that change have come other evolutions in medical interactions and practice, related mostly to the way doctors commu-nicate with you, record data about you, and share information with each other. Some of this is really good, and some is not. We'll explore that later.

But first, you might want to consider this: You probably know much more about the person who cuts your hair or your local bar-tender than the person charged with watching out for your health. I'd bet that if I polled people on how long doctors train to become practicing generalists or specialists they would be way off in their estimation. Six years? Eight years? The truth, depending on specialty, is more like 12 to 15. Let's see why this is so.

If we compare doctors to lawyers or accountants or other profes-sionals, we see that doctors spend more time in school than anyone else, period, full stop. With a few exceptions, there's 4 years of col-lege, 4 years of medical or osteopathic school (that's 8 so far), a year of internship (9 years), and then a residency of anywhere from 2 to 5 more years (11 to 14 years). There are even 1- or 2-year fellowships that can extend the educational process to the better part of a decade and a half. By the time many doctors get out of their training and actually see their own patients, they can be in their late twenties to early thirties. (I was an ancient 32 when I completed my anesthesi-ology program in 1989.)

Contrast that with lawyers who do 4 years of college and 3 years of law school—a piddling 7 years to argue about everything under the sun. Or 4 or 5 years max for an accountant. And I have not even mentioned the standard examinations one must pass—these are tests in addition to all the ones taken as part of the coursework for col-lege, medical school, internship, and residency. Aside from the typ-ical SAT or ACT test most every American student takes to enter college, the path in a physician's career involves the MCAT (medi-cal college admission test, taken during college), the three National Board of Medical Examiners exams (parts 1, 2, and 3, that lead up to licensure), and then the specialty board examinations. In my own case of the practice of anesthesiology, the board certification exam consisted of both written and oral examinations. You could not sit for the oral examination without first passing the written one. This is also the case in other specialties. And if that was not enough, there exists movement to require *re*certification in some specialties every 10 years or so, the so-called MOCA (maintenance of certification in anesthesiology) issue that has been raging in the courts. It's no wonder people are rethinking whether they want to do the long med school haul these days.

And then there's the debt. According to credible.com, 8 out of 10 medical school graduates borrowed an average of $251,600 to earn their degrees (often at high interest rates) and 18% of the students had borrowed $300,000 or more. The same website estimated that the average time to repay medical school debt was 13 years. When you consider how old you are when you finish your training, a doctor might be close to or over 40 years of age when that debt is repaid. That represents an increase of 97% when compared to debt during 1999–2000.

If that's not enough inducement to rethink medical school, consider the hours spent in training. Despite laws designed in the past few decades to limit interns' and residents' hours working, the Accreditation Council for Graduate Medical Education capped a workweek for medical house officers (interns and residents) to 80 (!) hours. This same organization set a limit to on-call frequency to no more than one every third night, a 30-hour maximum straight shift, and a minimum of 10 hours off duty between shifts. Yes—that's 30 hours working without sleep, rest, a change of clothes, or a shower. It has been noted that participation in this by training programs is voluntary, with violators subject to losing accreditation. "In my day," as us old-timers like to say, it was much worse. There were no such limits imposed on on-call frequency, hours per week worked, or rest between shifts. Even with the present system, life for a medical, surgical, or obstetrical intern or resident, and other types of interns and residents, can be exhausting and miserable.

And what can trainees in medicine expect as compensation for this 80-hour capped work week? According to Medscape's Resident Salary and Debt Report 2019, the average pay rate for a medical resident was $61,200 a year (mine was less than $15,000 in 1984), an increase of 3% from $59,300 in 2018. For an 80-hour workweek, admittedly an outlier, that comes to $14.71 an hour, less than my 19-year-old son is making working at Target after school. For a more realistic 60-hour-a-week pay rate, that comes to $19.61 per hour. What a pay hike that is.

There's also the issue of continuing education. States, not the federal government, run the licensing boards for doctors. Therefore, each state sets a standard for how many hours of continuing medical education is required per year (or 2 years in some states) to maintain licensure. Certification exams, the exams that designate a practitioner as a diplomate of a certain specialty board, is another issue. It used to be that a doctor would take this exam once and be certified for life. Then there was a move by some boards to have the doctor recertify every 10 years or so, depending on the specialty board. That has been fought against by many doctors in the courts as too onerous a standard to have to bear, and the doctors seem to have prevailed. This is an ongoing source of conflict and strife.

If you survive your medical training and have enough money left to get married, buy a house, and have some kids, then you should congratulate yourself. The bright side is this: According to merrithawkins.com, the 2019 Review of Physician and Advanced Practitioner Recruiting Incentives revealed a salary range for physicians of $239,000 a year, all the way up to $648,000 per year. The top earners were invasive cardiologists ($648,000), orthopedic surgeons

($536,000), gastroenterologists ($495,000), urologists ($441,000), dermatologists ($420,000), and anesthesiologists ($404,000). The lowest earners were family medicine doctors ($239,000), pediatricians ($242,000), internal medicine doctors ($264,000), and hospitalists ($268,000).

Clearly, doctors still command much higher salaries than most other professional groups. But is the stress, hard work, and sacrifice worth it? The answer lies not in the money but elsewhere.

According to BlackDoctor.org, doctors were the top suicide category among workers, with a 1.87 times more likely suicide rate than the average white American. They go on to note that whereas suicide is responsible for about 2% of all deaths in the general U.S. population, 4% of all physician deaths are self-inflicted. Dentists came in at number two (with a 1.67 times higher rate), followed by financial planners (1.51 times the rate), and lawyers (1.33 times the rate).

The high suicide rate among doctors is reflected in a proclivity toward substance abuse, although the abuse rate for doctors (somewhere between 10% and 15%) is said to be no higher than the general population of workers. However, the incidence of prescription drug abuse, as opposed to "street drugs," is much higher among doctors. The specialties with the highest rate of drug abuse among physicians were anesthesiology (my own specialty), emergency medicine, and psychiatry. This is not surprising, given the high stress associated with those areas of medicine and the fact that drugs are close at hand, a kind of "kid in the candy store" scenario.

The divorce rate among doctors is actually lower than in other professions—about 24%. The highest rate of divorce was seen in female physicians. It's not clear why doctors divorce at a lower rate.

I've often wondered what compels people to become doctors. Surely, as was true in my own career, a role model or models have a lot to do with it. My father was a doctor and my mother an operating room nurse. Many of my colleagues in medical practice relate similar stories. Then there are those people who have a fascination with science. Altruism plays a large role, as does the promise of a high salary and prestige.

But whatever the reason, it is very difficult for anyone to understand the heavy price to be paid who hasn't "been there"—anyone who hasn't dissected a cadaver stinking with formaldehyde, delayed his or her personal life and a decent income, incurred enormous debt, had the pleasure of working two full days straight without rest (and then doing it all over again two days later, then two days after that, etc.), seen people suffer and die, or lived under the nagging threat of litigation and the whims of reimbursement from the government and "third-party payors." I'm not looking for sympathy here, and after you have the physician income range I listed, you might not be inclined to offer it. Neither am I asking for your charity. I'm just suggesting you try to understand that becoming a doctor and practicing medicine is a grueling, stressful, and painful affair. The ugly and sad things we see as doctors can never be unseen, as is often the case with policemen, firefighters, and soldiers, and that exacts a toll. It makes some doctors prone to developing a thick skin, a detachment that lets them do their job and survive. That's something few doctors will ever tell you. Like soldiers who have seen battle and the horrors of warfare, most of us really prefer not to talk about it.

When I practiced clinical medicine, from 1984 to 2019, I learned I had to keep a lot of people happy. First, there were the patients and their families because, after all, you folks are always at the center of this circus. Then there are the administrators, the people who supposedly oversee the quality of our work and our practice habits. Then there are the folks at the state board of medicine, many of whom give not a whit about how long or carefully you have practiced—once you come across their radar, watch out! After that comes our insurers, the people who underwrite us for malpractice. And speaking of that, there are the plaintiff's attorneys, always a fun bunch to deal with. Add your own group's officers to the pile of characters as well. Then, of course, there's the federal government, which is always on the lookout for how you or your office manager "code" (recognized and predetermined billing language) for the procedures and diagnoses you submit for payment. Ditto for the insurers who, if the patient is not on Medicare or Medicaid or some other government medical program, have their own say about what they will and will not pay for. That's a lot of folks to satisfy, and it's becoming harder by the day.

Why harder? That's easy. Like never before, the private insurance companies (plus Medicare, Medicaid, and the rest of the people who tell most of us doctors what we can make) have their noses in our business. In theory, there's nothing wrong with that. The fox should not be guarding the henhouse. But ever since I heard my dad complain about the reimbursement process going back to when I was a kid in the 1960s, things seem to have gotten worse. "Metrics" was not even a word back then. Now that word and that horrible term "big data" are everywhere. Frequently, doctors have to meet certain predetermined care criteria to get paid, in whole or in part, for the work we do. That's not necessarily a bad thing, but there are some quite unfair aspects to this arrangement. Foremost on the list is that the American public, due to stress, sloth, and overeating, is chronically sicker than ever before. And that leads to worse patient outcomes, no matter how good the care given is. But doctors end up paying for that, whether it is their fault or not that a patient had a less than optimal outcome. That's just the way things have evolved. But hey, no profession is without headaches.

So what is the point in all this? I suppose it is to emphasize that doctors are first and foremost human, and that we make mistakes, can be less than kind or diplomatic, and have our share of stressors with which to contend. We should have never been put on a pedestal to begin with. But we are gradually being taken off that pedestal. A survey conducted in 1966 revealed that 73% of patients had "great confidence" in the leaders of the medical profession. By 2012, that number was reduced to 34%. I suspect it is still lower today. We most certainly are not supermen and superwomen. And I wish the general public, in light of the recent COVID-19 pandemic, would stop referring to us and other medical workers as "heroes." No one put a gun to our heads and told us we had to be healers. We cannot pick and choose whom we treat; our oath is to take all comers, whatever the risks, and do the absolute best we can. It was the same whenever leprosy or tuberculosis emerged, HIV became a thing, and hepatitis C was commonplace. All those conditions posed risks to practitioners, but we still had to be on the front lines, no matter what the consequences of exposure.

Still, patients expect a lot of their doctors. A Mayo Clinic study showed that when polled, patients said the "ideal" doctor should exhibit the following qualities:

- Thorough
- Empathetic
- Humane
- Forthright
- Confident
- Personal
- Respectful

Like Boy Scouts, doctors are expected to be prepared and on their best behaviors. Anything less is clearly not ideal.

Still, we keep you waiting long times in the waiting room. Not because we want to, but because we are strapped for time. According to a recent report from the NIH, one-sixth of a doctor's working time is spent on administrative duties, and this lowers their job satisfaction. Unlike in my father's time, we must answer emails and phone calls from patients, communicate with other physicians and consultants, keep our continuing medical education credits up to date, make sure our charts are dictated and signed, attend mandatory medical staff meetings, ensure that the codes we submit are accurate and (heaven help us) not construed as fraudulent, check lab reports, imaging reports and other tests—the list goes on. All of this takes attention away from you and other patients.

The other main stressor, as I have mentioned, is the constant fear of litigation. Although it "comes with the territory," malpractice lawsuits and their implications for doctors' careers and personal lives can be significant. (Did you know that surgeons leave behind, unintended, 6,000 surgical sponges, instruments, and other "retained foreign bodies" in patients each year?) On average, depending on specialty, doctors can expect to be sued every 7 years. And those who get sued have to wait years, in many cases, to know the outcome of the actions taken against them. Although insurance is supposed to cover and protect a physician's assets, there have been cases where the damages have exceeded the coverage limits, causing financial ruin for some doctors. Whether they deserved it or not, a physician's financial life and career can go up in flames with a hefty judgment or highly publicized case. The doctors who are at greatest risk for these high-profile and expensive cases—OB/GYN doctors, anesthesiologists, emergency room physicians, general surgeons, radiologists, orthopedic surgeons, and others—know full well that they are only as good as their last case or patient encounter. They realize that they are under constant scrutiny from the administrators, lawyers, state medical boards, malpractice insurers, and even their colleagues. Some deal with it better than others.

So next time you have a visit with one of your doctors, think a little about what you've read here. Yes, the odds are that your doctor makes more money than you. Oftentimes, much more. But think again: Would you really want to change places?

CHAPTER 7

First, Do No Harm

Medical Misadventures and Malpractice

Doctors, increasingly, are doing remarkable things. They transplant organs, devise pharmaceutical cocktails to battle cancer, separate conjoined twins, perform fetal surgery in utero while a woman is still pregnant, replace ailing or deformed heart valves though a tiny incision, and treat drug-resistant depression with magnets. They also screw up and harm patients. Big time. It has been estimated that the third-leading cause of death in our country is from the medical system itself—from medical errors committed *iatrogenically*.

The Greek word *iatro* means "physician," and anything good or bad caused by doctors is therefore iatrogenic. Sometimes iatrogenic results are benign, such as a small and insignificant scar left after surgery, or a minor side effect of a prescribed medication, like a temporarily dilated pupil in the eye. But whatever the clinical setting, an old dictum is consistently valid: *primum non nocere*. In a letter to the editor in the December 2001 edition of American Family Physician, a doctor wrote an article exploring the true meaning of the Latin phrase *primum no nocere*, or "first, do no harm." The editor of that journal commented in reference to the oft-quoted expression: "Try to help your patients when you can, and when you can't, at least try not to make things worse."

Whatever interpretation one might want to give, the sentiments expressed are similar to passages found in the famous Hippocratic Oath, where Hippocrates states:

> I will use my treatment to help the sick according to my abilities and judgment, but never with a view to injury. . . . I will . . . help the sick, and I will abstain from all intentional wrong-doing and harm, especially from abusing the bodies and man or woman.

Historically in medicine, there seems to be special attention paid to the crucial import, above all else, not to harm patients. Yet with the number of doctor–patient interactions reaching ever higher with each passing year, the number of prescriptions written, procedures performed, and surgeries inflicted grow as well, and the number of patients harmed in the crossfire rises at alarming rates. That's why, no matter what the economic conditions, whether in wartime or peace, or whether Republicans or Democrats in power, the malpractice plaintiffs' attorneys seem to always stay busy.

I used to get really angry about that, ever eager to portray that group of professionals with contempt. And even now, for those lawyers that continue to file lawsuits that are clearly frivolous and without merit, my contempt continues unabated. But my view has been tempered over the years the more I hear about how my medical colleagues and brethren have harmed patients. Much of that change in attitude came as a result of my professional capacity as an expert witness for both the defense and the plaintiff, for it was in reviewing the many cases that came to my attention that I came to learn of what we doctors can really do to harm people if we are not careful.

I began my medical school studies in 1979, but that's not when my medical education started. I had watched my dad endure the hardships and vagaries of medical practice since I was a small boy, going on rounds with him and listening to him talk on the phone with other doctors, pharmacists, and patients and their family members. From 1950 to 2007 my father treated and healed people.

His training was long and hard. First there was an internship and residency in New York City, then a fellowship at the NIH in Bethesda, Maryland. Then after a stint as an officer in the U.S. Public Health Service, he practiced endocrinology and internal medicine in the suburbs of Washington, D.C. Most every day he'd come home and tell me stories about this or that patient with such-and-such disease. The myriad medical journals lying around the house, complete with pictures and illustrations so gross and disgusting as to make me reluctant to even run my hand across the pages, overflowed from his bedside table. He'd be shaving in the bathroom adjacent to his bedroom and I'd read out, in broken and halting mispronunciations, the diseases from the articles in my hand, only to have him correct me and give a thumbnail discourse on the definition and nature of the condition in question. Years of all that were very illuminating.

When I finished residency and went out into practice, two things haunted me: "What if I hurt a patient? and "What if I get sued?" These nagging questions colored the way I looked at my own practice of medicine and my perceptions of the manner in which the physicians around me performed their duties. By the time my clinical career ended in 2019, I had seen enough of the good and bad in the practice of medicine to understand what really harms patients the most. Also, being a former director of risk management for a large managed care group rendered me arguably more astute than the average physician when it came to medical practice and civil law. Over the years, I developed a special interest in this area, and it was that interest and a desire for stronger patient advocacy that contributed to the writing of this book, as well as my monthly blogging on medicine, health, and healthcare.

All of that leads me to an examination of the errors that we doctors commit. The list is not meant to be exhaustive, just representative of the most common patterns and themes behind medical mishaps. Roughly, they fall into a few readily recognized categories:

- Communication shortcomings
- Unnecessary treatments and tests
- Incorrect diagnoses
- Administering the wrong medication
- Events that should never happen; in law, *res ipsa loquitur* cases ("the thing speaks for itself")
- Chasing the almighty dollar

The first category is so obvious yet so crucial. Communication breakdowns are a problem not unique to medicine, but medical practice lends itself to this type of error. First, doctors have notoriously bad handwriting. It's one of the oldest doctor criticisms around. Second, when many more specialists are consulting on patients than ever, there is bound to be a lack of coordination in care. Do the various doctors who write notes in your chart even read each other's opinions and comments? Are they checking to see that tests are not redundant or overordered? That medications are not duplicated or prescribed in a way that cause harmful interactions? That the order to stop or begin a new medication has been noted by all the relevant caretakers? That a urinary catheter, one of the major sources of in-hospital infection, should have been removed days ago? The advent of electronic health records has helped here, but it is not the entire solution.

Also, miscommunication doesn't only happen when practitioners fail to read the chart. It happens in all areas of medicine and in a variety of settings. A failure to communicate effectively doesn't just occur at sign-out rounds (where doctors, nurses, and other caregivers go over their patient lists and "hand off" care to the new on-duty team), by missing something written or recorded in the chart, or failing to follow up with the laboratory or radiology department.

I once knew of a case where a woman underwent a hysteroscopy in the operating room under general anesthesia. A newer device that measured the inflow and outflow of the irrigating fluid was being used during that procedure, but no one in the operating room appeared adequately trained (in the parlance: "in-serviced") in the use of that apparatus. Confusion related to the alarm system of the device and real-time troubleshooting its other uses ensued, and the operating room staff failed to tell the surgeon, who was focused on the surgical area, that the inflow and outflows of fluid were out of sync. The patient, who up until this time was under sedation anesthesia, rapidly developed pulmonary edema and an attempt at emergency intubation was made. But the intubation was unsuccessful because her face and airway had swelled so rapidly and severely from the excess fluid in her tissues. She had to have an emergency tracheotomy to establish an open airway and save her life. It was not my case—I just happened to pass the operating room and peeked in the window to see what all the commotion was about—but I did run and find the first general surgeon I could lay my hands on to perform the tracheotomy.

Unnecessary tests and treatments are an ongoing problem. In his 2014 book *Doctored: The Disillusionment of an American Physician*, Sandeep Jauhar writes:

> Overutilization in health care is driven by many forces: "defensive" medicine by doctors trying to avoid lawsuits (unnecessary tests add an estimated $150 billion each year to the health care budget); a reluctance . . . to accept diagnostic uncertainty (thus leading to more tests). . . .

Overtesting and overconsultation have become fact. . . . The culture today is to grab patients and generate volume.

The author goes on to describe how doctors have skirted the "kickback" rules of referral to each other and refashioned it into the "mutual scratching of backs." He says,

> Physician to physician referrals are doctors loudly declaring their independence from insurers and the federal government. . . . It is hard not to view a referral as an overture from another physician, and it is equally hard not to return the favor.

This increased calling in of specialists, which has risen from 5% in 2004 to 9% in 2014, can lead to more testing and prescribing, as well as creating more players in any one patient's medical drama. Sometimes two heads are better than one, but only if those heads coordinate with each other and are aware of the other's actions. The situation becomes more complex the more consultations are requested and the more specialists are involved.

Unnecessary tests can cause infection, unwanted radiation exposure, and a host of side effects. A spinal tap can give you a severe and persistent headache, sometimes only cured with the administration of an epidural blood patch. Intravenous dyes from radiologic imaging studies can lead to kidney failure and even anaphylaxis. Even a "routine" colonoscopy can leave you with a ruptured colon.

And then there's misdiagnosis. There are many causes for missing a diagnosis, not the least of which is the lost art of physical diagnosis. In my father's era, CAT scans, MRIs, and PET scans were just a dream. The clinician had to rely on careful history-taking, physical examination, and an interpretation of the existing laboratory capacities to formulate a diagnosis and treatment plan. Doctors of that day also had to have an *index of suspicion*, an attitude sorely lacking in today's medical world.

I have mentioned my late father, who practiced medicine from 1950 to 2007, and his habit of taking me on hospital rounds with him. He taught me a lot over the years about interacting with patients, physical diagnoses, disease states, and their treatments. But perhaps the greatest and most enduring thing he imparted was to always have an index of suspicion.

It was his former teacher, the legendary Isadore Snapper, MD, who taught him the same. Dr. Snapper, the former doctor to the Dutch royal family and a prisoner of war under the Japanese in World War II, was perhaps the greatest diagnostician of twentieth-century Western medicine. He was the master of so-called bedside medicine, a combination of art and science that relied mostly upon being an attentive medical detective. His colleague Hans Popper at Mount Sinai Medical Center in New York City where my father interned, said of him that he was "A physician for whom the word 'charisma' might have been invented." He taught his students that everything about the patient, from the way he/she looked, talked, walked, and even smelled, offered essential clues to diagnose and treat disease. But to get to even that point of diagnostic sophistication, required the clinician to care enough, pay attention enough, and have discipline sufficient to entertain all the possible reasons for what was evident from listening to and physically examining his or her subject.

Currently, I am that afraid this valuable but time- and energy-consuming practice is being lost. Today, doctor's attentions are diverted toward what the healthcare industry glibly calls "metrics," a garbage-bag term that encompasses everything from lab results, outcomes, vital signs, admission rates to hospital, days in the hospital, infection rates—you name it. Doctors today, who are taught to rely on diagnostic studies and lab results more than they ever did before, have largely lost this art of diagnosis that Snapper so brilliantly advocated, nurtured, and taught.

A visit to your doctor is more likely now to be a hurried affair, with your healer clacking away at a computer while you discuss your problems. Larger patient volumes, a by-product of our aging and sicker populace, is partly to blame. But so too is the reliance on test results and a deficient focus in medical education, so different now than in decades past.

Does this mean that people get less effective and satisfying treatment? I'm not sure. I cannot seem to find definitive evidence one way or another. But I will tell you this: Interventions, such as CT scans, X-rays, blood tests, and many more—too large in number to note—are driving costs up and do come with side effects. In many cases, a shotgun approach to diagnosis, in the worst scenario, replaces actually examining and listening to the patient. With this, the essential index of suspicion, that extra mile of thought and evaluation of the physical and spoken evidence a patient renders, is often lacking or even nonexistent. Let's be frank: Physicians of the later generation were raised to expect instant gratification, more so than their predecessors. Also, with the gadgets and distractions they were raised with, they have, clearly, a shorter attention span. This is self-evident—just look around you.

Not harboring an adequate index of suspicion can mean missing what's there and seeing something that isn't. In the case of missing a diagnosis, media is replete with stories relating to a patient who went to the doctor complaining of one thing or another, only to be dismissed as a hypochondriac or complainer, and later found to have some dreadful disease. My hometown newspaper, the *Washington Post*, publishes a regular column entitled "Medical Mysteries." Every time I read that section of the paper I am amazed and disturbed how often patients who go to untold numbers of doctors are shuffled around, dismissed, misdiagnosed, and even harmed. And there's a flip side to that.

An attorney friend from Boston told me of a recent case in which a man underwent a pancreatic biopsy and was told he had cancer. The poor man underwent a Whipple procedure, a notoriously long, involved, and sometimes dangerous surgery, only to be told later that the pathologist misdiagnosed the specimen and that the entire surgical ordeal was unnecessary. The man did not have cancer after all. But now he was rendered diabetic because the surgery removed a great deal of the insulin-producing cells in his pancreas. Stories of overdiagnosis and unnecessary and harmful procedures and testing abound.

I'm sure you're aware of a misdiagnosis or overdiagnosis tale in your own social circle or have read about it or heard a story on television or in other media relating to this all too common medical error.

Horror stories abound about patients receiving the wrong medication or the correct one in dangerous amounts. One famous case involved a child who received multiples of a standard chemotherapy medication dose and died as a result. Sound-alike drugs, like Xanax and Zantac, Pitocin and Pitressin, and Tramadol and Trazadone, can be confused and interchanged when phone calls are made or orders are dictated, resulting in catastrophes.

And then there are the *res ipsa loquitor* cases, the kind of legal torts that "speak for themselves," so egregious are their nature. These are the cases where a forceps is left behind in a surgical patient, the wrong limb is amputated, the wrong organ removed, the wrong patient is transfused blood or a mismatched blood transfusion is given to a patient, the wrong patient is operated on, and so on. My attorney friend says to the responsible party's insurer regarding monetary damages in these cases: "Take out your checkbook, write a '1' and then some zeroes. I'll tell you when you can stop writing the zeroes."

These are not the only categories in which errors occur. I have seen pure greed skirt that scenario—here is how. A few years back, I accepted an anesthesia assignment to cover a GI endoscopy practice, where gastroenterologists performed sigmoidoscopies, colonoscopies, and upper endoscopies. Almost everyone is familiar with colonoscopies (and the uncomfortable "prep"), the seemingly too frequent examination of your colon with the use of a flexible fiberoptic scope. Perhaps a fewer number of patients have undergone upper endoscopy, where the doctor looks into your throat, esophagus, and stomach using the same type of equipment.

Typical of that clinic was the scheduling of many cases during the day. There was one doctor in particular who booked an inordinate number of patients—19 to be precise—for the day, many of them double procedures (colonoscopies and upper endoscopies). We would begin the day at 7 am, go without a break until 6 or 7 pm and do a total of between 25 and 30 procedures on those 19 patients. By the time he and I reached the late afternoon, both doctors (myself and the GI doctor) and staff alike were not at their best. Although I managed to cover that assignment many times without any complications or medical mishaps, I swore to myself that I would never accept an assignment like that again. No doctor, however skilled and dedicated, will get away with such a grueling day for an extended time frame and *not* have an eventual mishap due to fatigue, inattention, or just plain carelessness. And that wasn't the only setting where this occurred. I've covered similar settings for 20 or more cataract surgeries, laser procedures, and other types of interventions where money was apparently the main driver in such an unreasonable and unsafe clinical construct.

No matter the root cause of medical mishaps, I tell you about them to be aware of them, be watchful for them and to protect yourself, as much as you are able to do so, from becoming a victim of the flaws in the system. Throughout this book, I try to give practical advice about how to best go about that. But make no mistake, errors occur at any time and place in medicine. Be careful. It can be dangerous out there.

CHAPTER 8

Time's Up

A Look at How We Die

While still in the midst of the COVID-19 pandemic that has claimed so many lives, gutted economies, and ruined the plans and health of many people, the United States suffers on with its traditional killers. So much attention has been paid to the ravages and fallout from the novel coronavirus that the other ways in which we die have, for now, been relegated to the back burner. But I am quite sure that after the virus that swept the world is long gone, the more "traditional" shopping list of the grim reaper will retain its primacy.

The leading killers, according to estimates from the CDC's mortality data for 2018, as well as some key related data, were reported by authors Jiaquan Xu, MD, Sherry Murphy, BS, Kenneth Kochanek, MA, and Elizabeth Arias, PhD. The ten leading causes of death for that year were unchanged from 2017. They were:

1. Heart disease
2. Cancer
3. Unintentional injuries

4. Chronic lower respiratory diseases
5. Stroke
6. Alzheimer's disease
7. Diabetes
8. Influenza and pneumonia
9. Kidney disease
10. Suicide

In 2017, the CDC reported 2,813,503 deaths in the United States. Heart disease was responsible for 647,257 deaths, cancer 599,108, injuries 169,936, chronic lower respiratory disease 160,201, stroke and cerebrovascular disease 146,383, Alzheimer's disease 121,407, diabetes 83,563, flu and pneumonia 55,672, kidney disease 50,633, and suicide 41,173. Of note was the fact that unintentional injuries was the leading cause of death in people ages 1 to 44.

Tellingly, an article in *USA Today* from October 24, 2018, by reporter Kate Morgan revealed a great overlap between the biggest killers and the most common afflictions that Americans suffer, which are:

1. Hypertension (high blood pressure)
2. Major depression
3. Increased blood cholesterol
4. Coronary artery disease
5. Type 2 diabetes
6. Substance abuse
7. Alcohol abuse
8. Chronic obstructive pulmonary disease
9. Psychosis
10. Crohn's disease and ulcerative colitis (inflammatory bowel disease)

The first leading cause of death in the United States should come as no surprise. Throughout this book I have spoken of Americans' terrible diet, physical inactivity, expanding waistlines, and the negative effects of stress and cortisol. Yet the hundreds of thousands of deaths every year from cardiovascular disease maintain its number-one status, year after year; it dwarfs the deaths from the COVID-19 epidemic. Observers who point that out are often quickly criticized by many as being rash or insensitive to the plight of the people who succumbed to that infectious disease. "Wait a minute," they say, "how can you compare heart disease to an infectious disease? It's like comparing apples to oranges!" Perhaps. But there might be more overlap than one might see at first glance. To me, poor health habits are "infectious" in the sense that bad habits "spread"—through advertising, the process of normalization, and societal expectations—reflected in bad diets and sedentary workplaces. Look at football tail-gating, with its fatty and greasy meals, overflowing with beer and sugary drinks. Memorial Day, the Fourth of July, and other public holidays often encompass the same. In everyday life, much of our lifestyles involve rushing to work, wolfing down unhealthy food, and stressing about bills, "appearances," and material things. Isn't that contagious in a sense? After all, it is what most everyone else is doing, is it not? During the wintry "holiday time" in America, when people pack on the pounds, rush around to chase material things, and basically neglect themselves and their bodies, only to vow to change their habits with the coming of the New Year, there is unmistakable and apparent groupthink when it comes to these activities. Media and Madison Avenue tell you what you must buy, how you should entertain, and what you should eat during that unnecessarily stressful time of year. If those attitudes aren't "contagious," I don't know what is.

That cancer deaths are a close second to heart-related deaths should surprise no one either. We are living longer, and with an aging population it is inevitable that diseases of older people, such as cancer, will kill more of us. We are also exposed to more toxins in our air, water, food, and soil than at any other time in human history. According to the National Cancer Institute, new cancer cases in 2020 most commonly involve lung, colorectal, pancreatic, and breast cancers, which are responsible for nearly 50% of all deaths from cancer. The lead cancer killers are lung and bronchus (135,720 deaths), colon and rectum (53,200), pancreas (47,000), breast (42,000), and other types (327,800). An estimated 606,250 people died from cancer in 2020. The article mentioned that cancer was responsible for 21.3% of all deaths in 2017, and that cancer and heart disease cause nearly half the deaths yearly in the United States. It is the leading cause of death for people under age 65.

Despite the scary numbers, cancer deaths are down nearly 30% in recent years. As Shawn Radcliffe recently reported on healthline.com, better treatments for four major causes of cancer (lung, colorectal, breast, and prostate) and a falling smoking rate have much to do with the decrease. Also, the death rate from melanoma has witnessed the most profound decline. During the period 2013 to 2017, melanoma death rates fell about 7% per year, contrasted with 1% to 3% during 2006 to 2010.

A lot of the decrease in death rates, as reported in the same article, were due to immunotherapy and other targeted treatments. The HPV vaccine has been instrumental in reducing cancers caused by human papilloma virus infections, which are related to cancers of the cervix, mouth, anus, and throat.

But whatever the cause of cancer, the author states "you can reduce your risk for many cancers by maintaining a healthy weight, exercising regularly, eating a healthy diet, avoiding all forms of tobacco and limiting alcohol intake." In other words, embracing habits foreign to the average American.

Unintentional injuries and chronic lower respiratory infections kill far fewer Americans than cancer and heart disease, partially because of wearing seatbelts and the significant reduction in tobacco abuse.

Death from cerebrovascular disease and stroke has fallen as well, mainly due to better blood pressure control, diabetes management (a disease that can contribute to higher stroke rates), blood lipid lowering, and lower smoking rates. But there persists a geographical predilection in our country for stroke, or CVA (cerebrovascular accident), in a region known as the "stroke belt" or "stroke alley." Like "the Bible belt," this area of the nation encompasses the southern states of Virginia, North and South Carolina, Georgia, Mississippi, Alabama, Kentucky, Tennessee, Indiana, Louisiana, and Arkansas. Northern Florida's and Texas's membership are debated. Incidentally, the CDC in 2011 sited research that the stroke belt overlapped geographically with the "diabetes belt," encompassing many of the same counties in these states. There has even been an association with these same regions and high rates of lung cancer.

Theories abound as to why the rate of stroke is higher in the counties of these states, areas with a peak incidence of stroke in the coastal regions of Georgia and South Carolina. Poor diets (heavy with fried and oily foods, refined starches, and sugar), poverty, maternal prenatal malnutrition, higher rates of tobacco abuse, a rural healthcare model (where access to quality healthcare may be restricted or unavailable), untreated hypertension, and disparities in ongoing treatment for those who have suffered a heart attack have all been proposed as reasons for the phenomenon.

Even the population density of African Americans in these states has been named as a factor. In their 2018 editorial in the online journal *Physiology*, authors Heidi Lujan and Stephen E. DiCarlo discussed the theory that blacks may have more prevalent and severe hypertension than other groups from genetic and environmental causes. They state:

> During a May 2007 Oprah show, Dr. Mehmet Oz asked Oprah "Do you know why African Americans have high blood pressure?" Oprah promptly replied that Africans who survived the slave trade's Middle Passage (slave ship journeys) "were those who could hold more salt in their bodies."

Presumably, the retention of blood sodium was genetically advantageous to surviving the grueling and water-restricted hell that was the experience of all who were forced to endure the slave ships from Africa. The authors open the article from a quote from Norman Kaplan and Ellin Lieberman from 1994 in the sixth edition of *Clinical Hypertension*:

> A very attractive case can be constructed, all based on a genetic defect in sodium excretion that is more prevalent among blacks. Perhaps blacks, who originally lived in hot, arid climates wherein sodium conservation was important for survival, have evolved the physiologic machinery which protects them in their original habitat but makes it difficult to handle the excessive sodium they ingest when they migrate.

This theory has been reported in the lay press many times before, and the authors of the online *Physiology* article are quick to refute it:

> The "slavery hypertension hypothesis" has gained prominence in the popular press and is often cited. The hypothesis is also highlighted in medical textbooks and taught in

many medical schools. However, we posit that the theory is not supported by the data . . . and should not be taught or promoted.

Whether valid or not, many who study stroke and cerebrovascular disease in the stroke belt are quick to note the African-American connection. It remains a point of controversy for sure. What is not controversial is the hellish history of the slave trade and the immoral, cruel, and inhumane treatment that the African slaves received in all aspects of their plight.

I have covered extensively the role of diet, physical inactivity and the resultant obesity epidemic, and the increase in diabetes in the West and developing countries. Naturally, this growing concern consistently appears on the top ten list of killers in the United States. Interestingly, I have many personal connections and brushups with this disease: My father, who suffered from it for most of his adult life, was a diabetologist. My sister succumbed to it at the young age of 26, having had all the severe complications from its juvenile form. And it was my dad's mentor, the great Isadore Snapper (who I reference elsewhere in this work) who first noted that the diabetic residents of China did not have nearly the severity nor range of complications from their disease than their American counterparts. He attributed this to a different diet in China, one that did not cause the neuropathy, kidney disease, loss of eyesight, and other complications we see in our own country. Because one in three Americans are deemed "prediabetic," we clearly have not gotten a handle on reducing the prevalence of this scourge.

Flu and pneumonia kill a lot of people, and the reasons for that are not hard to deduce. We are living longer, and those diseases are particularly lethal in older, debilitated people—the same people, aside from the younger "cytokine storm" victims, who lost their lives and suffer in the present COVID-19 pandemic.

Chronic kidney disease from any form, whether as a result of poorly controlled blood pressure, diabetes, vasculitis (inflammation of the blood vessels) or other autoimmune and more unusual causes, is the ninth most deadly killer. Dialysis and transplantation have been seminal in keeping people with the most serious cases of renal insufficiency alive, but those interventions come with a heavy price, physically, emotionally, and financially. Chronic dialysis is a complicated and unpleasant undertaking: Transplant patients must stay on immunosuppression drugs the rest of their lives.

The tenth most common killer is suicide, whose stigma, along with emotional illness in general, I discuss elsewhere in this book. There is overlap among the top ten categories (kidney disease can come from hypertension and diabetes, pneumonia from COVID-19, etc.) and this last one is no different. There has been much written about "death of despair," an area of social and medical research that deals with the lower life expectancy of middle-aged white Americans, starting around 1998 and culminating in 2014. Many investigators have looked at this issue and the conclusions are variable. In the March 23, 2020 edition of the *New Yorker* magazine, physician author Atul Gawande postulated that economic factors were paramount in this entity. In analyzing the research of two Princeton investigators, he found that the recurrent themes of job loss, chronic pain, drug addiction (partially related to the then-raging opioid epidemic), depression, physical illness, availability of firearms, and low economic growth for uneducated whites in middle-age lead to an alarmingly high rate of suicide and earlier death than their cohorts in other ethnic and racial groups. Combined with self-inflicted death from other populations, we can see why suicide is a serious problem in our country. It is unlikely, given the current political, social, and economic climate, to improve anytime soon.

CHAPTER 9

"Say Again?"

The Secret Language of Doctors

Physicians, like soldiers, policemen, lawyers, accountants, and other professionals, speak a secret language. Their arcanum is based primarily in Latin and Greek and relies heavily on well-recognized prefixes and suffixes that have a formula all their own. Doctors also speak a second language, a slang complete with abbreviations (more on that later), that evolved over many years and was made known in popular culture by the 1978 novel *The House of God*, by Samuel Shem. Much of the words, attitudes, and clinical perspectives of that book have fallen out of favor over the years—and we should be thankful for that. But there are still remnants of those antiquated attitudes, and even newer and at times more biting slurs and phrases, that still creep into the informal medical lexicon.

Patients who have perhaps a greater degree of freedom and power over their medical records and what is contained in them, compared to the realities extant in 1978, often express confusion and ignorance when trying to make sense of their medical charts and history, Depending on the policies of the doctors' offices, insurance companies, or health plans they deal with, patients have varying degrees of access to what they can read about themselves medically. A patient's chart is not merely a compilation of diagnoses and treatments. It includes, in its full form, test results (blood, urine, spinal fluid, and other work on bodily fluids and emissions), imaging studies (X-rays, CT scans, MRIs, PET scans, ultrasounds, and the like), consultants' reports, and a host of other information.

Often this information is fragmentary, although there have been advances, with the advent of consolidated medical records, to codify a person's written and visual medical history. Many patients do want to know what is said about them medically, but not all patients have full access to what the doctors might see. One important exception to this is the case of the malpractice, or medical lawsuit, where lawyers get to pore over what doctors oftentimes would rather not be made public.

But lawsuit or not, patients enjoy more access now to their medical histories, as recorded by doctors and other healthcare workers, than perhaps at any time in modern history. And most people would say that's a good thing; it allows for transparency, candor, and even the ability to attempt to correct errors in the record that could have costly implications—say, for procuring life insurance and other purposes. Some people just want to know what healthcare people have written about them. Others want the information for their record-keeping. Still others are merely curious. Whatever the reason, unless you are in the medical business, you probably won't understand a lot that is written about you. That's where this chapter comes in. I want to give you a way to navigate and understand what is being said about you medically, from a basic standpoint. This is not an introduction to medical school, just a method of deciphering medical terms, abbreviations, and jargon.

Crucial to an understanding of medical words and terms is to realize that they are based mostly on roots or derivatives of Latin or Greek, two languages that doctors have used to treat patients over the centuries, before English, French, Russian, German, or any other modern language got involved in medical education. That's not to say that these languages abandoned the Latin and Greek roots of medical terminology. To the contrary. The persistence of these terms is a testament to the strength with which medical professionals have clung to the "classical" foundations of the language of the healing arts.

There's really nothing magical to medical language. Most of it, based on a prefix and a suffix, is easy to grasp once you have the translation key. For example, two of the most common prefixes in medical talk is *hyper*, meaning "too much of," and *hypo*, meaning "too little." Thus, *hyperthyroid* literally means "too much thyroid," and *hypothyroid* means "too little thyroid" (referring to the function of that endocrine gland). Hypertension, or high blood pressure, is easily understood in this context, as is hypotension, or low blood pressure. Similarly, the prefixes *micro-* and *macro-* mean "small" and "large," respectively. *Microcephaly* means "small head," and *macrocephaly* the opposite. *Microcytosis* means "small cells," and usually refers to small red blood cells. *Macrocytosis* means "large cells."

When I was first released onto the wards of Boston City Hospital as a third-year medical student on July 1, 1982, I was bewildered by the terminology that I found in the chart. It was bad enough that I had, up to that time, minimal if any clinical experience where I would actually lay hands on a patient. When instructed by my intern to review the chart of Mrs. So and So, I read something like the following:

This is the 2nd BCH admission for this 45 YO WF with CC: "my stomach hurts."

HPI: The patient is a 45 yo wf who presents to BCH ER with CC of RUQ pain. The pain has been there 2 months and gets worse after eating a fatty meal. PMH is sig for

HTN, obesity, NIDDM and RA. She had NKDA. She is a 20PY smoker. She is 18 months s/p RIH hepair.

Her meds include HCTZ, metformin and Indocin.

On PE she is a middle aged WF, obese, in NAD.

P 77 R 20 T 98 BP 143/88 Ht. 5'6" W 213

I was totally lost. If someone had given me the keys to translating this mess, I would have at least noted the following:

This is the 2nd Boston City Hospital admission for this 45-year-old white female with chief complaint: "my stomach hurts."

History of present illness: the patient is a 45-year-old white female who presents to the Boston City Hospital emergency room with chief complaint of right upper quadrant pain. The pain has been there for 2 months and gets worse after eating a fatty meal. Past medical history is significant for hypertension, non-insulin-dependent diabetes mellitus and rheumatoid arthritis. She has no known drug allergies. She is a 20-pack per year smoker. She is 18 months status post right inguinal hernia repair.

Her medications include hydrochlorothiazide, metformin, and Indocin.

On the physical exam, she is a middle-aged white female, obese, in no acute distress.

Pulse 77, respirations 20, blood pressure 143/88. Height 5'6" weight 213.

But no one ever had given me the keys—"the keys" to translating this double-talk and gobbledygook. That's why I'm giving you the keys here and now.

Understanding medical talk is easy once you learn the basic terms. Prefixes fit with suffixes in any number of ways. If you are old enough to remember when Chinese restaurant menus asked you to pick one item from column A and one from column B, the same applies to medical prefixes and suffixes.

For anatomic terms, starting from the head to the toes, the following prefixes apply:

- cephalo-: pertaining to the head
- cranio-: the skull
- facial-: the face
- cortico-: cortex of the brain
- cerebello-: the cerebellum
- oculo- or ophtho-: the eyes
- oto-: the ears
- naso-: the nose
- oro-: the mouth
- esophago-: the esophagus
- pharyngo-: the throat
- tracheo-: trachea or windpipe
- dento-: the teeth
- fascio-: the connective tissue
- gingiva-: the gums
- lingulo-: the tongue
- cervico-: the neck
- thyro-: the thyroid

- brachio-: the arm
- carpal-: wrist
- pectoro-: the chest
- cardio-: the heart
- musculo-: the muscles
- osteo-: the bones
- chondro-: the cartilage
- mammo-: the breast
- pulmono-: the lungs
- broncho-: the air passages
- alveolo-: the air sacs
- lympho-: the lymph glands
- hepato-: the liver
- spleno-: the spleen
- gastro-: the stomach
- entero-: the intestines
- choleo-: the gallbladder
- dermato-: the skin
- umbilico-: the navel
- inguino-: the groin
- reno-, pyelo-, or nephro-: the kidney
- ano-: the anus
- recto-: the rectum
- vagino-: the vagina
- oophero-: the ovaries
- salpingo-: tubelike
- utero-: the uterus
- vesico-: the bladder
- phallo-: the penis
- testiculo-: the testicles
- onycho-: the nails
- tricho-: the hair

- mano-: the hand
- pedo-: the foot
- digito-: the finger or toe
- femero-: thigh
- tibio-: shin
- patello-: kneecap
- tarsal-: ankle
- onycho-: the nails
- adreno-: the adrenal glands
- pancreatico-: the pancreas
- duodeno-: the duodenum
- uretero-: the ureter
- urethro-: the urethral
- audio-: hearing
- visuo-: seeing
- colo-: colon
- ileo-: ileum
- cecal-: cecum
- neuro-: nerve
- cyto-: cell
- arthro, rheumatic-: the joints
- erythro-: red
- leuco-: white
- thrombo-: platelet
- megalo-: big
- micro-: small
- onco-: cancer
- sub-: below
- supra-: above
- infra-: within
- inter-: between
- thoraco-: chest

- lumbo-: lumbar, lower back
- sacro-: sacral
- coccygeal-: tailbone
- sarco-: flesh
- a-: absence of
- antero-: the front of
- posterio-: the rear of
- uni-: one of
- bi-: two of
- tri-: three of
- quadri-: four of
- multi-: many
- hydro-: pertaining to fluid

This list is not exhaustive, but it does represent the most common prefixes that pertain to anatomy, relevant descriptors and body parts, diseases, and disorders of organs and systems.

And now the suffixes.

- -ology: the study of
- -osis: pertaining to that organ or system
- -itis: inflammation of
- -emia: in the blood
- -uria: in the urine
- -biliary: in the bile
- -dynia: pain of
- -graphy: recording of
- -algia: pain
- -ectomy: removal
- -gram: recording of
- -lysis: destruction of
- -oma: swelling

- -otomy: incision or hole
- -phagia: eating or ingesting
- -phasia: speech
- -philic: attracted to
- -plakia: plaque-like
- -rhea: flow of
- -plasty: surgical repair of
- -oscopy: to examine with an instrument
- -stasis: equilibrium of
- -trophy: growth of
- -thermia: pertaining to temperature

Constructing and deciphering medical terms, with certain rules and exceptions, is easy when combining prefixes and suffixes. You can try it yourself from the two preceding lists. Again, consider it like choosing from column A and B from a Chinese restaurant's menu. *Pancreatitis* means "inflamed pancreas." *Macrocytosis* means "large cells." *Arthroplasty* means "joint reconstruction." *Gastroenteritis* is "an inflamed stomach and intestines." And so on.

There are web references and books available to expand upon these lists and that also deal with the minutia of the rules about properly constructing the terminology. But what I've presented here should give you a basic start in your ability to translate terms in your chart.

The abbreviations are another matter. They have evolved over the decades and indeed are constantly changing as medicine and technology have changed. Here are some you might come across:

- WDWN: well-developed, well-nourished
- NAD: no acute distress
- PE: physical exam
- CC: chief complaint

- HPI: history of present illness
- FH: family history
- PERRLA: pupils (eye) equal, round, reactive to light and accommodation (distance)
- WM, WF: white male, female
- AAM, AAF: African American male, female
- CHF: congestive heart failure
- CVA: cerebrovascular accident, stroke
- TIA: transient ischemic attack, mini-stroke
- MI: myocardial infarction, heart attack
- GSW: gunshot wound
- ETOH: alcohol
- IVDA: intravenous drug abuse
- PE: pulmonary embolus, lung blood clot
- RA: rheumatoid arthritis
- DJD: degenerative joint disease
- ARF: acute renal failure
- CRF: chronic renal failure
- NTG: nitroglycerin
- RHD: rheumatic heart disease
- SL: sublingual (under the tongue)
- CAD: coronary artery disease
- CABG: coronary artery bypass graft
- AVR: aortic valve replacement
- MVR: mitral valve replacement
- NSR: normal sinus rhythm
- LVH: left ventricular hypertrophy
- RVH: right ventricular hypertrophy
- LAE: left atrial enlargement
- RAE: right atrial enlargement
- ECMO: extra corporeal membrane oxygenation
- HNP: herniated nucleus pulposis

- DM: diabetes mellitus
- IDDM: non-insulin-dependent diabetes
- TKR: total knee replacement
- TKA: total knee arthroplasty
- CCK: gallbladder removal
- THR: total hip replacement
- I and D: incision and drainage
- BMI: body mass index
- OSA: obstructive sleep apnea
- CPAP: continuous positive airway pressure
- DOA: dead on arrival
- Appy: appendectomy
- TURP: transurethral resection of the prostate
- STD: sexually transmitted disease
- SAT: blood oxygen saturation
- PFT: pulmonary function test
- BP: blood pressure
- P: pulse
- RR: respiratory rate
- T: temperature
- ARDS: acute respiratory distress syndrome
- SIDS: sudden infant death syndrome
- T and A: tonsillectomy and adenoidectomy
- D and C: dilation and curettage
- TAH BSO: total abdominal hysterectomy, bilateral salpingo-oopherectomy
- BKA: below-the-knee amputation
- CTR: carpal tunnel release
- ACL: anterior cruciate ligament
- PCL: posterior cruciate ligament
- PTSD: post-traumatic stress disorder
- Bx: biopsy

- Dx: diagnosis
- Rx: treatment
- Cx: cancellation
- PPI: proton pump inhibitor
- CT, CAT scan: computerized axial tomography
- MRI: magnetic resonance imaging
- PET scan: positron emission tomography
- S/P: status post (after having had a procedure)
- IV: intravenous
- ICU: intensive care unit
- CCU: coronary care unit
- ER: emergency room
- NICU: neonatal intensive care unit
- PICU: pediatric intensive care unit
- GA: general anesthesia
- SDH: subdural hematoma
- SAB: subarachnoid block, spinal anesthesia
- C/S: caesarian section
- PPD: purified protein derivative
- TB: tuberculosis
- AMA: against medical advice
- DNR: do not resuscitate
- AF: atrial fibrillation
- SR: sinus rhythm
- VF: ventricular fibrillation
- V tach: ventricular tachycardia
- SBE: subacute bacterial endocarditis
- PFO: patent foramen ovale
- AR: aortic regurgitation
- MR: mitral regurgitation
- MUGA: multigated acquisition (scan)

- PEEP: positive end expiratory pressure
- COPD: chronic obstructive pulmonary disease
- GERD: gastroesophageal reflux disease
- ASH: asymmetric septal hypertrophy
- MS: multiple sclerosis
- MND: motor neuron disease
- PCO: polycystic ovaries
- SIADH: syndrome of inappropriate antidiuretic hormone secretion
- PY: pack years of smoking cigarettes (yrs. times packs per day)
- URI: upper respiratory infection
- A line: arterial line
- SG catheter: Swan Ganz catheter, to measure circulatory pressures
- PVC: premature ventricular contraction
- PAC: premature atrial contraction
- PE: physical exam
- NPO: nothing by mouth
- QD: each day
- TID: three times a day
- BID: twice a day
- QID: four times a day
- QHS: at bedtime
- QAM: in the morning
- PO: by mouth
- PR: by rectum
- ECCE: extracapsular cataract extraction
- IOL: intraocular lens
- NG: nasogastric
- ETT: endotracheal tube

Now that you have the essential language tools of medicine, you are prepared to translate, on a basic level, what healthcare providers are saying about you or someone you care about. Should this matter to you? Maybe it doesn't. But if you are, as I suspect, like a growing number of people who want to take better control of their health and the information said about them, then it would behoove you to familiarize yourself with the prefixes, suffixes, and abbreviations I have presented.

Of course, just being able to read the terms and abbreviations is half the battle; the interpretation is what is important. I trust that some of the material presented in this book, combined with the information in this chapter, will assist you in making sense of your medical record. This is important and valuable. I will tell you why.

First, it benefits you and helps your doctor to verify the accuracy and timeliness of your medical record. Maybe you lost 40 pounds and no longer are on blood pressure medicine. If that is true, good for you. You should be proud of yourself. However, it should also be reflected in your chart, where the diagnosis "hypertension" can be taken off the list. This will also help ensure that you are not continued on any unnecessary therapy, like blood pressure medicine, as patients often are when a diagnosis changes and the veracity of the record suffers when details slip through the cracks in the healthcare sidewalk.

Second, an understanding of your record gives you the power to make better decisions on what areas of your health to focus on. It helps to see what's listed first, covered most extensively, and what conditions have been studied, treated, and counseled on the most. If there are a lot of cardiac issues addressed in your record, for example, you can see what tests have been done, what results have been recorded, which therapies have been prescribed, and your doctor's impressions about the effectiveness of your care plan.

Third, the sicker you are, it seems, the more you pay in life insurance and other policies. It would be of great benefit to you financially to make sure your medical record is accurate and up to date. You shouldn't have to overpay for something that is not supported by fact.

Fourth, being medically literate empowers you to do more and better things about your health. If your record keeps reflecting visits and interventions related to one diagnosis or condition more than others, you know you can work more on that, as I have said earlier. But the literacy you have gained can do more; it can get you thinking that the secret language of medicine does not have to shut you out as an active participant in maintaining your most important asset. You do not have to be intimidated by the jargon written about you. You can read your chart, formulate your own questions, and make more informed and cogent decisions about your health. Once the veneer of intimidating, lofty, and puzzling medical language is stripped away, you can decide what habits to adopt and what goals to set to improve your health.

I encourage you to keep a copy of this book with you when you go for a medical visit. That way, the terms and abbreviations will be readily available for you to refer to. It will also show your healthcare provider—whether physician, nurse, physician's assistant, therapist, or other caretaker—that you care enough to want to *really* understand what they are saying about you. You can ask to see notes from your PCP (primary care physician), specialist, or others and ask intelligent questions about what the information means and what you can do to make the situation better. This will impress your caretaker, no doubt, and may lead them to treat you with more careful attention and respect.

CHAPTER 10

Mini–Med School, Part 1

A Primer of Form and Function

With the wealth of information instantly available to most people through the use of a computer, mobile device, or other web-access technology, it is astounding that many patients simply haven't the first clue about how their body works and what the instructions from their healthcare providers actually mean. Writing on health illiteracy in an August 2011 article on the website governing.com, reporter Tina Trenker had this to say:

> Technically, health literacy is defined by the U.S. Department of Health and Human Services (HHS) as "the degree to which individuals have the capacity to obtain, process, and understand basic health information and services needed to make appropriate decisions." The percentage of the U.S. population who can do so is shockingly low. Only 10 percent are fully literate when it comes to health instructions, according to HHS's Office of Disease Prevention and Health Promotion (ODPHP).

Nearly 15 percent are totally health illiterate, mostly due to language barriers.

In between those extremes, around 40 percent of the adults in the U.S. have only "basic" or "below basic" health literacy levels. People with basic health literacy have trouble deciphering clearly written pamphlets explaining, say, medical testing. Those with below basic literacy have trouble with forms of all sorts, and with basic directions for taking medication.

The human cost is telling. . . . Low health literacy is linked to higher rates of disease and mortality, as many as 100,000 deaths per year. Among all adults—regardless of age or nationality—low health literacy adds up to more frequent use of hospital emergency rooms and inpatient care, and a much lower likelihood that people will follow through on basic preventive measures. . . .

The ODPHP estimates that limited health literacy runs the nation between $106 billion and $236 billion annually. . . ." the ODPHP report says, "the real present day cost of limited health literacy might be closer to $1.6 to $3.6 trillion."

These sobering sentiments regarding the medical illiteracy of the American public has been echoed elsewhere, with even more dire statistics. The U.S. Health and Human Services Office of Disease Prevention and Health Promotion has found that a mere 12% of adults in our country possess adequate health literacy. This has meant that those patients who cannot fathom basic medical information are, according to studies, at higher risk for being admitted to the hospital and are less likely to use preventive health services. Clearly, this lack of essential primary knowledge costs individuals and society both personally and financially.

If you are reading this book, you are likely more informed, more curious, and more interested in maintaining or improving your health than the average American. But I wonder—How would *you* perform on a basic test of health and medical knowledge? Here goes:

1. The lymphatic system is primarily related to:
    A. A network of nerve cells that dictate the automatic functions of the human body
    B. Organs and channels that help clear toxins and waste products from the body
    C. Ligaments that help organs stay in their proper position
    D. The filtration of ingested liquid to form urine
2. The organs responsible for calcium balance in the body are located in the:
    A. Head
    B. Neck
    C. Chest
    D. Abdomen
3. True or false: All arteries take oxygenated blood away from the heart and to the rest of the body.
4. Hemoglobin, the molecule that carries oxygen in the blood, is dependent on what element as part of its structure and proper functioning?
    A. Copper
    B. Magnesium
    C   Iron
    D. Calcium

5. Medicare was primarily formed to help:
   A. Low-income people with health insurance
   B. Hospitals build new infrastructure
   C. Senior citizens get adequate health coverage
   D. States access the health records of their government employees

6. True or false: The air we breathe is almost entirely made of oxygen.

7. The largest organ in your body is your:
   A. Skin
   B. Liver
   C. Vascular endothelium (blood vessel lining)
   D. Brain

8. If you had to, you could live as an adult without which of the following organs?
   A. Brain
   B. Liver
   C. Heart
   D. Spleen

9. If you receive a prescription that says to take a pill t.i.d., how often should you take it?
   A. Every six hours
   B. Every 12 hours
   C. Every 8 hours
   D. Once a day

10. An EEG test measures:
   A. Brain waves
   B. Heart impulses
   C. Breathing function
   D. Muscle strength

11. People with inadequate kidney function are known to have high levels of what in their blood?
    A. Creatine
    B. Creatinine
    C. Iron
    D. Hemoglobin

12. Morbid obesity places a person at higher risk of:
    A. High blood pressure
    B. Diabetes
    C. Degenerative joint disease
    D. Acid reflux disease
    E. All of the above

13. Body mass index is a rough estimate of:
    A. Muscle strength
    B. Flexibility
    C. Foot and hand size
    D. Healthy or unhealthy body weight

14. Ideally, general anesthesia means that:
    A. Surgical patients are numb from the waist down only
    B. Surgical patients are partially awake for their operation
    C. Surgical patients are unconscious and unaware of their surroundings during surgery
    D. Doctors can bill much more for their services

15. True or false: These days both an M.D. (doctor of medicine) and a D.O. (doctor of osteopathy) can get privileges at most American hospitals.

16. What is the traditional sequence of medical study in the United States?
    A. Medical school, college, residency, internship, and fellowship
    B. College, medical school, internship, residency, and fellowship
    C. Residency, medical school, internship, fellowship
    D. Medical school, fellowship, residency, and internship

17. An intravenous allows healthcare providers to:
    A. Give much-needed fresh air to the lungs
    B. Drain the urine from a patient's bladder
    C. Administer fluids and medication to the patient's circulation
    D. Lubricate the patient's joints

18. Rheumatology is the medical specialty that deals primarily with:
    A. The brain
    B. The joints and connective tissues
    C. The intestines
    D. The ovaries and uterus

19. True or false: Americans are now living longer than ever.

20. People who get addicted to narcotic medicines are:
    A. Almost always minorities
    B. Almost always poor
    C. Prone to this addiction due to painkillers prescribed to them after surgery
    D. Unlikely to be found among the wealthy in our society

Here is your answer key: 1. B, 2. B, 3. False, 4. C, 5. C, 6. False, 7. C, 8. D, 9. C, 10. A, 11. B, 12. E, 13. D, 14. C, 15. True, 16. B, 17. C, 18. B., 19. False and 20. C.

I wonder how you scored. I hope not too badly, but I would not be surprised if many of you did not do that well. If that is the case, you are clearly not alone. That is what this book and this chapter are all about. Throughout this book I have attempted to give you essential, succinct knowledge that will help you make better decisions about your health and well-being. In this chapter, I would like to give you a basic medical primer—a "mini-med school" of sorts—to augment your basic understanding of human structure (anatomy) and the way your body works (physiology). The value in this is elementary: Once you grasp the basics of the structure and function of your most prized possession, your organs and tissues, you can understand how and why it is so important to incorporate habits that keep these parts of you working as best as they can, despite your genetics and your environment.

I am mindful that I risk insulting your intelligence, and I certainly do not mean to. But it is a fact that even highly educated people lack the basic understanding of the way their bodies work and how the diagnosis and treatment of medical problems are accomplished. I am often taken aback in discussions with academics, lawyers, business folks, and professionals of all stripes by their relative paucity of medical and healthcare knowledge. I was shocked recently when a close friend, who teaches at Princeton University, asked me what a CAT scan was. Ditto when seemingly educated friends refer to the male sex gland behind the bladder as the "prostrate" or that they just underwent a "colonostomy" to look for colon polyps.

I'd wager if you put an interviewer on a busy street corner in New York City and had him ask passersby the question "Why do people need to breathe?", other than receiving some strange looks and a few snarky remarks, he might hear "To get air into your lungs." And if the interviewer asked a follow-up question of "Why is that important?" he might hear "Because we need oxygen to live." But then, if you would ask "Why do we need oxygen to live?" not one in a thousand people would be able to tell you that oxygen is needed because it is essential, through the biologic metabolic pathway known as oxidative phosphorylation, in the production of ATP (adenosine triphosphate) through the transfer of electrons in the cell. It is ATP, the organic compound produced as a by-product of oxidative phosphorylation, that renders the energy necessary to run the many and complex processes of cells, as well as act as a building block to DNA and RNA. So without oxygen, there is no oxidative phosphorylation, no ATP, and no life.

That might get one in a thousand people thinking, I would hope, that the lungs that breathe air (which is 20.9% oxygen), transferring the contained oxygen to the blood traveling through the lungs, and the heart that pumps the oxygenated blood to every tissue and cell in our bodies (through oxygen both dissolved in the blood and attached to hemoglobin in the red blood cell) are crucial to life and should be cared for, nurtured, and cherished. These organ systems—the lungs, the heart, and the arteries, capillaries, and veins—are unfortunately on the front line of the abuse we mete out through poor health habits. We smoke, vape, and breathe polluted air, which hinder our lungs' ability to take in oxygen effectively. We strain our heart and vascular systems with poor diets, lack of physical effort, and chronic stress, thus blocking our arteries, clamping down our blood vessels, and tearing up the lining of these delicate and essential internal roadways.

Surely, most grade-schoolers know that brains think, hearts pump, lungs breathe, stomachs digest, muscles contract, eyes see, and ears hear. But perhaps fewer numbers comprehend that kidneys filter, livers detoxify, and glands secrete hormones essential for crucial life functions. However, aside from early efforts to become educated in these areas, it appears that, for people not involved in medical care, the interest in anatomy and physiology wanes. It is usually not until an individual, a family member or friend, becomes ill that there resurfaces the potential interest in wanting to know what is going on, and that is a shame. Because if more people learned the basics, we would all be better off for it.

You could approach an understanding of the workings of your body a number of ways. You might start from the head down, listing each organ, its structure, and its function. You also might take a "systems" approach, describing say the "circulatory system" or the "digestive system." Another possibility is to approach it from a medical specialist's point of view by examining the purview of the cardiologist, the gastroenterologist, the dermatologist, and so on. All of these approaches have their plusses and minuses. But instead of getting tangled up in unnecessarily long and involved anatomic and physiologic discussions, it's best to look at the three lists I have referenced earlier in this book—the top ten medications, the top ten supplements, and the top ten killers—to gain the most practical understanding of the workings of your body. Only then can you get at the real "meat" of medical intervention: addressing pathophysiology.

The prefix *patho-* refers to "abnormal," and when applied to physiology the resultant term *pathophysiology* is merely a fancy word for what we called at my medical school in Boston "the biology of disease." But before we embark on our primer of pathology as it relates to the most commonly seen ailments in our society, let us first take a basic look at the anatomy and physiology—the form and function—of what makes us human beings.

Almost all humans share basic physical characteristics. Aside from genetic predispositions and recognized congenital syndromes, we come, like new cars off the lot, with the same "standard" equipment: one brain, spinal cord, nose, mouth, tongue, esophagus, stomach, small intestine, large intestine, appendix, thyroid gland, liver, bladder, spleen, pancreas, sex organ, uterus (female), prostate (male), and two eyes, ears, nostrils, lungs, arms, legs, hands, feet, testes, ovaries, kidneys, and adrenal glands. We are all covered with skin, have bones and muscles that provide us with scaffolding, ligaments and tendons to hold it all together, a vascular system for our blood, a network of nerves that allows electrical impulses to coordinate voluntary and automatic (autonomic) functions, and a microanatomy (histology) within our specialized organs where all the real work is done. With the tens of trillions of cells that make up our bodies, it is truly a miracle that anything goes *right* with it.

But we risk getting too involved here unless we stick to our purpose: to gain an elementary understanding of our form and function. Let's start at the top and work our way down.

Our skull, that bony covering that has our jaw (or mandible) attached to it, houses our brain. The outer layer of the brain, the cerebrum, is its biggest part and allows for reasoning, sensation, speech, memory, learning, and emotional and fine motor control. Behind and below the cerebrum is the cerebellum, responsible for coordination of movement, balance, and our unique posturing abilities. The brainstem, residing below the cerebrum, is the nervous system's "Grand Central Station," acting as a relay nexus for the brain and spinal cord. Many autonomic functions that we take for granted, including temperature regulation, heart rate, breathing, wakefulness, and others, are controlled through nerves and nuclei (concentrated collections of nerve cells) that emanate from the brainstem.

On our way down the body, two major organ systems reside one in front of the other: the pulmonary and digestive systems. We intake the air we breathe through our nose and mouth, where it enters the trachea. The tracheal pipe (our windpipe) splits at the *carina*, a structure in our central chest that leads to our two mainstem bronchi. As the pulmonary tree divides into smaller and smaller airway passages, eventually these conduits lead to the *alveoli*, the tiny air sacs that are covered by innumerable tiny capillaries. It is there that the crucial exchange of gases (oxygen and carbon dioxide) between the air sacs and the bloodstream take place. We extract oxygen from the air we breathe and excrete carbon dioxide (CO_2) when we exhale.

Your heart, having four chambers (two atria or auricles and two ventricles), is about the size of your fist. It is perfused by the *coronary arteries*, the blood vessels that often get occluded (blocked) by cholesterol plaques. The aorta, arising from the left ventricle, is the main artery to the body. This superhighway gives life-sustaining oxygen-rich blood to the cells and tissues of the body. The pulmonary artery arises from the right ventricle and passes oxygen-poor and carbon dioxide–rich blood to the lungs, where at the alveolar/capillary interface, the blood dumps off its carbon dioxide waste and extracts oxygen from the air we breathe.

Your heart has a sophisticated electrical conduction system that is responsible for coordinated pumping of your atria and ventricles. Two rhythm stations—the SA node (sinoatrial node) and AV node (atrioventricular node)—are specialized tissues that are responsible for proper cardiac electrical conduction and the heart beating. Two other specialized cardiac muscle fibers responsible for your heartbeat, *the bundle of His and the Purkinje fibers*, also play a role in optimal heart rhythm functioning.

With regard to your all-important vascular endothelium (your largest organ), I refer you to Chapter 2 of this book to review its essential form and function.

Positioned behind our respiratory system is the upper part of our digestive system: our mouth, tongue, esophagus, and stomach. After digestive enzymes and our tongue break up our food into a manageable size, we swallow the food and deliver it via our esophagus to our stomach. Further digestion takes place there before the products of digestion are delivered lower down to our small and large intestines, structures that have their own unique purposes. The small intestine, about three times the length of your body, is where the vast majority of nutritious elements from your digested food are absorbed into your bloodstream. Recent studies have highlighted the importance of your small intestine in mood and sleep through the actions of the neurotransmitter serotonin. The bacteria within your small intestine, its microbiome, may also serve an important role in regulating your immune system.

Your large intestine, comprised of your cecum, colon, and rectum, is about 6 feet long. Its purpose is to rid the body of the waste left over after all the nutrients from the food we ingest has been extracted. It is also crucial in water and electrolyte absorption, and has a microflora of its own that is important.

There is an expanding science exploring the *gut-brain axis*, the connection between the intestines and the central nervous system whose importance is still being explored. Talk about your "gut feeling"—there you have it.

The *endocrine system* (pertaining to internally excreting glands) is to be found throughout the body and is to be distinguished from the *exocrine system* (externally excreting glands). Endocrine glands is the collective name given to the structures that release hormones, which travel to the tissues and cells of the body to effect certain changes that are essential to life. These hormones govern a variety of key body functions, including our emotional state, growth, symmetric development, specific organ function, procreation through sexual function, and metabolism. The endocrine system from head to toe includes the following: the hypothalamus, the pineal gland, the pituitary, the parathyroids, the thyroid, the pancreas, the adrenal glands, the ovaries in females, and the testes in males. Briefly, the glands do these things:

- **The brain's hypothalamus.** Tells the pituitary what to do through chemical messengers in the blood. Gathers information from the brain on the environment, including temperature, light intensity, and sensations.
- **The brain's pituitary.** The "master gland." Makes prolactin (to enable breastfeeding), corticotropin (which tells the adrenals

what to do), growth hormone (for growth of all the bodies tissues and bones, as well as the body's utilization of minerals and ingested material), antidiurectic hormone (which regulates water balance), oxytocin (which causes uterine contraction in childbirth). This gland also influences sex hormone production in the reproductive organs and the secretion of the "feel good" chemical known as endorphins.

- **The brain's pineal gland.** Releases the sleep-regulating hormone melatonin.
- **The neck's thyroid gland.** Makes chemicals that dictate metabolism, as well as control heart rate, body temperature, skin composition, and mood.
- **The neck's parathyroids.** Embedded in the thyroid gland. Help control body calcium levels.
- **The adrenals.** Two glands, one atop each kidney. Have an outer part, the cortex, that makes corticosteroids, essential for electrolyte and fluid regulation and the body's response to stress, reproductive capacity, and even the immune system. The inner part, the medulla, makes epinephrine (also known as adrenaline) and other stress chemicals, which control blood pressure and heart rate.
- **The testes and ovaries.** The testes make testosterone, which turns boys into men, physically. The female gonads, the ovaries, produce estrogen and progesterone, which are important in female bodily development, the menstrual cycle, and pregnancy.
- **The pancreas.** Where the blood sugar–controlling chemical insulin is made by the *islet cells*. It's located in your abdomen not far from the lower part of your stomach.

Doctors who deal with diseases of the gastrointestinal tract also study conditions of the liver, the abdominal organ found on the right side of your body in what doctors call the right upper quadrant. This detoxifying organ also has roles in metabolism, bile production, hormone synthesis, and the breakdown of erythrocytes (red blood cells). This organ is so prolific in function that it has been estimated by scholars to serve about 500 functions.

Your spleen is a large organ in your lymphatic system, located on the left side of your body between your 9th and 11th ribs, and is important for fluid regulation and helping your immune system stave off infections. Adults can live without their spleens; they are important in children for development of a fully functional immune system.

Your kidneys are crucial for so many functions, such as filtering toxic wastes and water from your blood and producing urine. They are central in the production of hormones that help form red blood cells. They also regulate blood pressure and bone metabolism. Urine is produced when liquid waste is passed from the kidney to the bladder by way of the ureter. When the bladder sends a signal to the brain that it is time to urinate, the bladder contracts and expels the urine through the urethra and out of the body.

It is beyond the scope of this book to discuss the form and function of the remaining structures of the human body (your skin, reproductive system, skeletal and muscular systems, details related to your sensory organs, etc.), but information about the basics can easily be found on the internet using any number of reputable websites. One that I have mentioned before, which is unique in actually seeing how things work, can be found at www.blausen.com. I highly recommend the content found there.

Before we move on to pathophysiology—the ways in which things go wrong with our bodies—it is useful to note the ways medical professionals assess how well (or ill) you are. These methods unfold in a historical and logical sequence, reflecting medical progress in their increasing sophistication and complexity.

From the time of the first physicians, the patient's story or *history* and physical findings or *examination* were the only methods available to diagnose disease. Though still essential today, these methods, which depend heavily upon the inclination and skill of the investigator, have taken a back seat to laboratory tests, imaging studies, and more advanced methods of detection and diagnosis. This is too bad, because with these more modern methods have come a reduction in both the teaching and application of the arts of history-taking and physical diagnosis. Some medical schools don't even use real cadavers for their anatomy course now, resorting to online images of cadavers and other representations of the human body. Part of this is due to the difficulty some schools have in procuring deceased persons' bodies for study. Apparently, other schools like to teach anatomy without the real McCoy present. I am sure somebody somewhere has studied the differences in the two teaching methods, but I am not aware of any that show a difference in didactical outcomes.

Ancient physicians did things no doctor would consider doing today: tasting their patient's urine is one of them. Today, with the capabilities inherent in modern medical practice, there is ample ability to draw upon any number of testing modalities. I am certain the vast majority of people reading this book will have undergone some if not most of these diagnostic interventions: blood and urine testing, sputum and cerebral spinal fluid analysis, conventional X-rays, CAT scans, MRIs, PET scans, sonograms, electrocardiograms, electroencephalograms, pulmonary function tests, cardiac stress tests, coronary angiography, venograms, arteriograms, MUGA scans (a radioactive tracer test for heart function), and others. Some of these come with little or no side effects or risk. Others do carry risk, as well as discomfort. That is why it is so important to discuss the cost–benefit analysis for most of the tests your doctor orders for you. And remember this: Because they are available and because we love to waste things in this country, doctors are often quick to order more tests than are necessary. And waste is not the only factor. The practice of "defensive medicine" to avoid a medical malpractice suit is another clear reason why doctors are sometimes so test-happy.

This is not to imply that these lifesaving modalities are not without merit. The longevity we enjoy today is due in large part to these developments. However, keep in mind a central message of this book: Yes, we are living longer, but we are living lives dominated more and more by chronic illness, some more manageable and less burdensome than others. If we just changed a few of our more egregious behaviors, our improved longevity would be accompanied by, and rewarded with, a better quality of life.

CHAPTER 11

Mini–Med School, Part 2

A Primer of the Biology of Disease

By examining these top ten lists I mentioned, you are able to see patterns in human "Western" pathophysiology. Diseases of the heart, circulatory system, lungs, brain, and central nervous system, and cancer, which can affect multiple organ systems, stand out, as do the medications and supplements that treat those illnesses. Probing how and why these patterns emerge is the most effective way to teach the pathology (biology of disease) section of my "mini–med school."

Let's start with the heart and circulation. In Chapter 2, I described the vascular endothelium as the body's largest organ, and a chemically active one at that. Because much of what is important in the physical structure of human beings is merely plumbing (think blood vessels such as arteries, and veins and tubes such as the ureter, urethra, bile duct, and fallopian tubes), pathways and networks (nerve bundles, the spinal cord, peripheral nerves), and scaffolding (bones, joints, tendon, ligaments, and muscles), the blood vessels and heart are a good place to start. Your heart is a muscle supplied with its own oxygen-delivering arteries: the coronary arteries. These are the arteries that get bypassed or stented when blockages threaten their health and longevity. This pump has to last you a lifetime and gets so much abuse. The arteries that feed and nourish the heart muscle get clogged with plaques, which are fatty deposits that develop in some people through a combination of unlucky genetics and poor health habits. In a similar way, the arteries, the outflow pathways by which the heart carries life-giving oxygen to all the tissues and cells of your body, carry the blood that completes its oxygen transport and pickup of carbon dioxide at the cellular tissue level by means of the capillaries, the tiny vessels that form the billions of networks in every corner of your body. I am keeping it simple for a reason, but for those of you who want to learn more about the transfer of oxygen and pickup of carbon dioxide at the cellular level, look up the aforementioned term *oxidative phosphorylation*. You will have plenty to read.

The health of the heart and circulation (your arteries, veins, and capillaries), which themselves are dependent upon oxygen delivery to the blood by way of the lungs, is essential for existence. Factors that negatively affect both the ability to take in air and the delivery of oxygen by arterial blood to tissues and cells are reflected in so many common illnesses. The removal of CO_2 from those same structures by way of venous blood back to the heart (and then to the lungs, where the CO_2 is exhaled) is just as important. Remember, the body excretes carbon dioxide as a waste product of metabolism and takes in oxygen to nourish the tissues and cells to enable life. Any restrictions or imbalance to these equations lead to illness.

First on the oxygen-uptake side, the lungs can be impaired— whether from asthma, emphysema, chronic bronchitis, scarring, pulmonary fibrosis, edema, or any number of usually man-induced conditions—in their ability to transport the oxygen in the air we breathe to the pulmonary (lung) circulation. For it is oxygenated blood from the lungs that gets carried back to the heart and then out to the rest of the body by way of the left ventricle and then the aorta.

But even if the bellows (i.e., the lungs) are working fine, the pump (i.e., the heart) needs to live up to its end of the deal. Remember, if the plumbing to all the body or the heart itself gets clogged with fatty deposits, bad things may happen: The block might occlude blood flow, or a clot may partially break off (embolize) to obstruct blood flow to a vital area, such as heart muscle or a portion of the brain. In the latter case, this can cause a stroke, a term that relates to an interruption of oxygen-rich blood to the brain, whether from a clot (embolus), blockage (plaque), or hemorrhage (broken blood vessel).

This is why diet, exercise, and genetics are so important to circulatory health. We humans mess with this system in any number of ways. High blood pressure can cause the heart to work too hard, because it must pump against an increase in resistance. Like any machine that works too hard, it can compensate, fail, or die. One way it compensates is to have the muscles of the left ventricle, one of the four chambers of the heart responsible for pumping the blood out into the major highway to the body (the aorta), get bigger and thicker. This is called left ventricular hypertrophy, and when it develops, this can lead to more problems. Then, thickened heart muscle needs more oxygen to function, and blocked coronary arteries cannot keep up. This may, like in the case of any restriction to heart muscle blood flow, lead to a myocardial infarction (heart attack), where part of the heart muscle dies. Once that happens, some people are prone to developing heart failure, yet another complication of poor cardiovascular health habits. In some cases, that causes a backup of fluid in the lungs, leading to pulmonary edema, a condition where the lungs fill with fluid that had been forced out of the circulation from the plumbing system's back pressure.

The delicate interplay between blood flow to the heart, the restrictive pressure of too constricted, inflamed, and blocked arteries, the reduced oxygen delivery to the red blood cells in the lungs from the pulmonary ravages of smoking, air pollution, and primary lung diseases, all put people at risk for cardiovascular disease. But as we have seen, it does not merely stop there. The brain and other parts of the body, like the legs and other vital organs, can suffer from emboli (clots), blockages, and a lack of oxygen delivery from any number of sources.

It is easy to see why blood pressure and cholesterol-lowering medications are so commonly prescribed. Less common but still important pharmacologic agents related to thinning the blood (like the anti-inflammatory drug aspirin) to prevent clots, medicines to steady heart rhythms and improve the pumping capacity of the heart, and diuretics to remove excess fluid from the lungs when edema occurs are used as well.

But the tragedy is that so much of this illness could have been avoided with simple steps to address dietary and lifestyle issues. But again, most people do not even know the basics of anatomy and physiology enough to understand why their destructive habits, behaviors that come about by any number of bad reasons, lead to so much suffering. It is all too nebulous, too inconvenient, and foreign to the conscious mind, and after all, "What I don't know won't kill me, right?"

And what about the brain, that most complex and fascinating of structures. It too is heavily dependent on oxygen, as well as glucose, to function well and survive. I have already mentioned stroke, a major killer on our list of 10. But what about the brain's structure and its relationship to pathology? The brain is comprised of the cerebral cortex, where thought, speech, motor function, perception, and a host of other vital nervous system functions reside. There's the cerebellum, responsible for coordination of movement, and the limbic system (the hypothalamus, amygdala, thalamus, and hippocampus) system, where our emotions are housed. The thalamus is a way station to the cortex for sensory and motor transmissions, and the hypothalamus helps regulate body temperature and sends signals to the rest of the body via hormones. The hippocampus is involved in memory, among other things. The pineal gland is a mysterious small gland in the brain, thought to regulate both sleep and hormone levels, and the pituitary, the so-called "master gland" of the body, responds to signals from the hypothalamus to send hormones that regulate other organs as part of the endocrine system.

Many of these structures can become damaged from strokes, physical trauma (such as brain injuries related to contact sports and military-related trauma), toxic exposure, malignancies, infections, autoimmune illnesses, and other diseases. I mention them because so many people in our country suffer with diseases that impact these structures: multiple sclerosis (where the myelin "insulation" of nerves is damaged), Parkinson's disease (where the central supply of dopamine is reduced), depression and anxiety (where serotonin, norepinephrine, and other neurotransmitters are awry), schizophrenia, and Alzheimer's disease, just to name a few.

As important as the brain is, we cannot minimize the other components of the nervous system: the spinal cord and peripheral nerves. They too can be affected by many of the same factors that impair brain function. Part of these systems involve the 12 cranial nerves and the autonomic nervous system. The 12 cranial nerves, remembered by medical students for more than a century by the mnemonic "On Old Olympic Towering Tops, a Finn and German Viewed Some Hops" for the nerves olfactory, optic, oculomotor, trochlear trigeminal, abducens, facial, vestibulocochlear, glossopharyngeal, vagus, spinal accessory, and hypoglossal emanate from the brain and brainstem. These nerves dictate our sense of smell, our vision, pupillary reactions, sense of taste, eye movements, as well as other autonomic (sympathetic and parasympathetic) and movement functions. I mention them here because certain well-known diseases and conditions are associated with them. Trigeminal neuralgia is one of them. A very painful and debilitating condition, this disease (also known as tic douloureux) affects the trigeminal nerve and its ganglia in the brain. My dad suffered from it for over 40 years. Until medications and surgery were available to treat it, many of its sufferers committed suicide from the severity of the pain. The facial droop from Bell's palsy (often as a result of a viral illness), which affects the facial nerve, is also well-known to many. An acoustic neuroma is a noncancerous tumor that grows on the vestibular nerve and can affect hearing, cause tinnitus (ringing in the ears), and imbalance. I would bet you know at least one person who has suffered from one of these disorders.

Your autonomic nervous system dictates many "automatic" functions, such as the pace of your heartbeat, your digestion, body temperature, metabolism, sexual response, and so many more processes too complex for the scope of this book. I mention it here for the sake of completeness and to indicate that a variety of illnesses that affect nervous system function can impact the autonomic nervous system.

Two significant afflictions of the peripheral nerves—which allow for sensation, movement, and balance (proprioception) to your skin, deeper tissues, bones, and skeletal muscle—are diabetic neuropathy and multiple sclerosis. In uncontrolled diabetes, the chronically high levels of blood glucose have a negative impact on the health of your nervous system, including your peripheral nerves. Many people fail to realize that diabetes is not only a glandular (endocrine) disease, where the cells of the pancreas that make the hormone insulin are deficient or defunct, but very much a vascular disease as well. The small blood vessels that nourish the nerves can become damaged from long-standing poorly controlled diabetes, leading to the neuropathy that causes chronic pain, loss of sensation, and even an impaired sense of balance. In multiple sclerosis, the myelin lining of the nerves has been damaged. In this disease, the fatty coating (myelin) that assists in proper propagation of a nerve impulse has been attacked and altered in an autoimmune process. Both diabetic neuropathy and multiple sclerosis afflict millions of Americans, causing much suffering and disability.

Because diabetes treatments and mortality are so prominent on our lists, it is worth exploring the root causes of the disease in Western society. In general, it is fair to say that 100 years ago, when physical labor and easy access to "bad" calories was less prevalent, diabetes was not as much of a problem as it is today. According to an article in Diabetes.com.uk from January 15, 2019, the disease was first described about 1550 BC, where "an Egyptian papyrus mentions a rare disease that causes the patient to lose weight rapidly and urinate frequently." Note the use of the word *rare*. According to the 2017 CDC report "Long-term Trends in Diabetes," the disease has grown. In 1958, a mere 0.93% or 1.58 million people in the United States suffered from it. The numbers have surely and steadily increased: by 1975, 2.04% or 4.19 million people had it; by 1987, 2.77% or 6.61 million people; and by 2015, 7.40% or 23.35 million Americans had diabetes.

With about 10.5% of the population, or 34.2 million Americans, having diabetes today, we can see the severity of this condition's impact and scope. I have already discussed the root causes of this phenomenon throughout this book and will only mention the complications (the pathophysiology) that can arise from the most severe forms of the disease. The chronic excess of glucose in the blood and the impairment in blood flow in diabetics causes damage to what doctors call the "target organs": the eyes, brain, blood vessels, kidney, heart, and other structures and systems. My late sister, who died at age 26 from complications related to juvenile diabetes (insulin dependent, or type I), was blind, had a failed kidney transplant, suffered severe neuropathy (damage to the nerves, including motor, sensory, and autonomic), and had elements of an impaired digestive tract (gastroparesis) toward the end of her life. Indeed, on our top ten killers list, kidney disease is listed, and many of those cases are due to complications from diabetes. (Other causes of renal failure exist, most prominent among those is uncontrolled high blood pressure.)

Diabetes is a tricky disease to label and treat. There have been differing classifications over the years. Type 1 was traditionally associated with what was called insulin-dependent diabetes, and type 2 non-insulin-dependent (meaning, treated with pills or other measures). But many people who start as non-insulin-dependent diabetics end up on insulin. Some patients even take insulin and pills together. And it was not until recently, when medical science developed the research sophistication, that it was discovered that type 1 diabetes was actually caused by an autoimmune process. What is clear is that poorly controlled diabetes—as measured by some standard blood tests: the fasting blood sugar, random blood sugar, and the hemoglobin A1C test (HbA1C)—puts you at risk for all the complications my late sister had.

A normal fasting blood sugar, the test of blood glucose that is taken after an overnight fast, should be less than 100. A random blood sugar test, taken anytime during the day, should be less than 126. And depending on the laboratory, the HbA1C test, which measures how high your blood sugar is over many months, should be less than 5.8 to 6.0. Doctors also perform glucose tolerance tests (GTT), where you are asked to drink a sweetened beverage and then blood samples are drawn at intervals after the injection of the drink. If you are prone to developing diabetes or have the disease, the test will be abnormal.

General risk factors for developing diabetes are well-known: a family history of it, advancing age, obesity, a sedentary lifestyle, removal of the pancreas, and other causes places you at risk. That's why it is so important to consider the advice I have offered in this book and make your own decisions as to whether the changes I present make sense for you.

You may have heard about metabolic syndrome, a combination of disorders that place you at risk for cardiac disease, type 2 diabetes, and stroke. The combined characteristics, so common in today's population, are hypertension, elevated blood lipids (cholesterol and/or triglycerides), excess body fat (especially near the waist), and elevated blood sugar. Millions of Americans fit into this category, and many of them are heading for trouble. That is why it is so important to act now to prevent these terrible conditions from ruining your health and your life.

I have examined factors that impact your heart, circulation, lungs, nervous system, and kidneys, as well as touched on diseases like diabetes, multiple sclerosis, Bell's palsy, trigeminal neuralgia, acoustic neuroma, stroke, and heart attack. One separate category on the top ten killer's list is Alzheimer's disease, a condition that seems to be discussed and studied more and more with the passing of time. When initially categorized by Dr. Alois Alzheimer in 1906, it was described as a mental disease that affected memory and mood, and was responsible for other psychiatric disturbances. The cause of 60% to 70% of all cases of dementia, as the NIH website nia.nih.gov /health/alzheimers describes it, is:

> an irreversible progressive brain disorder that slowly
> destroys memory and thinking skills and . . . the ability to
> carry out the simplest tasks. In most people . . . symptoms
> first appear in their mid-60s.

Dr. Alzheimer discovered microscopic changes in the brain, eventually named neurofibrillary tangles and amyloid plaques, which were related to abnormal clumps of tissue. The website addresses the causes, which may include "a combination of genetic, environmental, and lifestyle factors." The writers went on to say there might be a relationship between Alzheimer's and cardiac conditions, stroke and hypertension, as well as obesity and diabetes. They conclude "a nutritious diet, physical activity, social engagements, and mentally stimulating pursuits have all been associated with helping people stay healthy as they age. These factors . . . might reduce the risk of . . . Alzheimer's." As you may have guessed, I could not have said it better than that myself.

The NIH's statement on the possible root causes and therefore the best prevention of Alzheimer's disease is in line with the basic tenets of this book: That lifestyle changes, particularly with respect to diet and physical activity, coupled with the reduction of stress and the development of meaningful relationships and stimulating activities, is your best health insurance policy.

Two top ten lists in Chapter 8 detailing the biggest killers and most common afflictions in America reveal a great deal of overlap. Both lists reference heart disease, diabetes, psychiatric issues, respiratory-related illnesses, and complications leading to stroke, such as high blood pressure and high blood cholesterol. But there were a couple of differences: namely cancer and inflammatory bowel disease. Cancer was the second biggest cause of mortality. Inflammatory bowel disease was listed as tenth in its impact on American health. But do realize that there is significant overlap and interrelationships between diseases. Diabetes can lead to stroke and kidney failure; hypertension, and the same autoimmune diseases, can predispose some people to cancer and so on. That's why it is so important to attend to your general health, for in doing so you protect yourself from developing any number of illnesses, as the NIH report on Alzheimer's disease stated.

No curriculum in our mini–medical school would be complete without examining the biology of disease related to the endocrine (glandular) system, cancer, autoimmune disease, and disorders of behavioral health (psychiatric disorders). In addition to the common conditions and killers that I have alluded to, these areas of concern make up the bulk of what destroys lives, taxes the already overburdened heathcare system, and eats up healthcare (and there-fore government) dollars.

Our discussion of diabetes was but one small aspect of diseases of the endocrine system, because any number of disorders can affect the endocrine glands described in the previous chapter. Many of them can become under- or overactive (through cancer or autoimmune pro-cesses), causing any number of predicted physiologic problems. Brain tumors, like a pituitary adenoma, can cause the pituitary to secrete too much hormone, resulting in headaches, changes in vision, and abnormal sexual function. Underactive thyroid, often a result of an autoimmune problem (Hashimoto's disease), can cause too little thy-roid hormone to be released, leading to fatigue, changes in bowel hab-its, feeling cold, hair loss, weight gain, depression, and other changes. Adrenal adenomas, which are tumors of the adrenal gland or glands, can lead to an overproduction of adrenal hormones and varying clin-ical disorders, such as blood pressure, weakness, and muscle cramps.

My point here is not to describe every disease that can arise in your endocrine system, but to point out that autoimmune conditions and/or cancers of any of these structures can give signs and symp-toms as to their presence and produce hormonal and other chemical alterations in your body that could make you even sicker.

You probably know someone who has had thyroid cancer, an under- or overactive thyroid, a pituitary tumor, cancer of the pancreas, testicular or ovarian cancer, or any number of other complications relating to these organs. Many famous people have suffered from this: Lance Armstrong with testicular cancer, Ruth Bader Ginsburg with pancreatic cancer, Gilda Radner and Elizabeth Montgomery with ovarian cancer, John F. Kennedy with adrenal gland insuffi-ciency, and the list goes on.

For the sake of completeness, I wanted to mention this impor-tant bodily system and make you aware of the different afflictions that are so commonly seen today. Even though many of these do not make our top ten lists, they are prevalent enough that you should be aware of them.

Which brings me to cancer and autoimmunity, two conditions that are often, but not always, interrelated. Interest in the causes, diagnosis, and treatment of diseases related to cancer and autoimmunity has never been greater, and enormous progress has been made in treatments for these conditions. It would be difficult to find any American whose life—personally or through loved ones or friends—has not been affected by cancer or autoimmune disease. The National Cancer Institute says that, based on data available from 2013–2015, about 38.4% of men and women will be diagnosed with cancer at some point in their lives. According to reports from Johns Hopkins University, autoimmune diseases strike about 3% of the U.S. population, or about 10 million people. Broken down, they say that autoimmune diseases impact people in descending order as follows:

- Hashimoto's thyroiditis: approximately 1,300 cases per 100,000 people
- Graves' thyroiditis: 1,100/100,000
- Rheumatoid arthritis: 875/100,000
- Vitiligo: 400/100,000
- Type 1 diabetes: 150/100,000
- Pernicious anemia: 200/100,000
- Multiple sclerosis: 100/100,000
- Lupus, Sjogren's syndrome, and myositis: less than 50/100,000

Women are affected more than men in all categories except type 1 diabetes.

It is important to note that about 1.3% of American adults suffer from some form of inflammatory bowel disease (either Crohn's or ulcerative colitis). The CDC says that this is an increase from 1999, where the statistics were 0.9% or 2 million adults. The risk factors for inflammatory bowel disease (IBD), according to the CDC report were:

- Aged 45 or older
- Hispanic or non-Hispanic white
- Less than high school education
- Unemployed
- Born in the United States
- Living in poverty
- Living in suburban areas

These numbers do not include people under 18. The report concluded that most IBD patients discover they have the disease in their 20s or 30s.

It is important to note that IBD is not strictly thought of as an autoimmune disease. WebMD states in a 2019 report that IBD "... has often been thought of as an autoimmune disease, but research suggests that the chronic inflammation may not be due to the immune system attacking the body itself." (Thus, its absence from the Johns Hopkins list.)

But whether cancer or autoimmune disease, these conditions make their presence too well-known in our lives. I like to think of them as criminals of two types: thugs and drive-by shooters. The "thug," cancer, used to be a model citizen until it became a "bad apple." Either through unlucky genetics or external mutation from viral, chemical, or other exposure, the patient's normal cells of a certain tissue "broke bad" and became deranged. Once deranged, this rogue cell multiplied like crazy, overtaking normal tissue and spreading its poisonous tentacles locally, and in the case of metastatic or invasive cancer, elsewhere in the body. Depending on the metastatic nature (aggressiveness) and the degree of derangement of the cell type (undifferentiated or poorly differentiated), these cells will consume much of the body's energy sources to stay alive and keep reproducing. That's why cancer is often such a "wasting" disease, where people lose weight and muscle mass. That's why any unexplained weight loss in an adult is particularly worrisome.

In the case of autoimmune disease, the drive-by shooter's victims are the patient's normal cells. In autoimmune disease, an immune response is mounted by the body's immune system (the drive-by shooter), which is activated to combat a "perceived" threat. The threat may not even be real (real threats could include bacteria, viruses, fungi, chemicals, or any other entities the body sees as not its own). In the process, the patient's normal tissues, like an innocent bystander, are attacked in the same or similar manner as the material that is seen as the foreign invader, which leads to possible organ damage and dysfunction.

Cancer therapy, an area of medicine that has changed immeasurably in the past decade, encompasses a range of treatments: surgery, chemotherapy, radiation (x-ray and proton beams), immunotherapy, bone marrow and stem cell transplantation, gene therapy, the list is growing. Treatments for autoimmune disease have advanced as well; the old standby of suppressing the immune response with steroids is still used, but there are newer treatments. As noted by uspharamacist .com, other standard drugs like methotrexate, cyclophosphamide, and sirolimus are being joined by more cutting-edge agents called "biologics" or biologic response modifiers (ending with the suffix -*ab*), as well as disease-modifying drugs (ending with the suffix -*cept*) that have shown promise in tempering autoimmune disease. In cancer care, there are newer drugs called immune checkpoint inhibitors, which the website cancer.gov describes as ". . . a type of drug that blocks proteins called checkpoints . . . made by some types of immune system cells, such as T cells, and some cancer cells. . . . When these checkpoints are blocked, T cells can kill cancer cells better."

Cancer and autoimmune diseases can be difficult to treat due to their complexity in diagnosis, staging (in the case of cancer), and implications for other organ systems of the body. For example, if lung cancer has caused much of the lung tissue to be removed, damaged, or destroyed, a pulmonologist will have to assist in optimizing whatever lung function remains. A patient whose pancreas has been removed for cancer will need the care of an endocrinologist to help manage the newly insulin-deficient patient's blood sugars. A person who lost a limb to bone cancer will need physical therapy and perhaps a prosthesis to live a better and more functional life. Patients with autoimmune diseases often get a delay in diagnosis due to the frequently vague and confusing cluster of signs and symptoms inherent to their diseases.

That is why it is so important to aggressively pursue the finest treatment for these conditions you can. Unlike a condition such as simple, uncomplicated hypertension, which is usually successfully handled by your own physician, cancer and autoimmune diseases are optimally treated at university-affiliated hospitals and medical centers. There, your chances of finding the newest and most effective treatments for your problems increase. Not every patient will have access to these centers, but it is important to seek it out to the best of your ability. Misdiagnosis and mistreatment in these conditions can be a real problem—don't be a victim of that if you can help it. Among the most commonly misdiagnosed diseases (according to an article written by Naveed Saleh, MD, in a June 4, 2020 article in MDLinx.com) are lupus, rheumatoid arthritis, and multiple sclerosis. The article claims that misdiagnosis is as high as 1 in every 20 patients, or about 12 million Americans. You can see why the stakes are so high when serious and complex diseases like cancer and autoimmune disease are among the differential diagnoses. Get second (and third) opinions if you are able. Be insistent and aggressive, but polite. Do your research and ask friends and family for help. These diseases are not to be taken lightly.

To better illustrate this point, consider this frightening example from the June 30, 2020 edition of the *Washington Post*. In its Health and Science section regular feature "Medical Mysteries," reporter Sandra Boodman told of a patient whose diagnosis of a rare type of blood cancer took 17 years to diagnose. A 31-year-old man and athlete was complaining of lack of energy, painful wrists and ankles, and was found to be anemic. He had consulted numerous doctors, including neurologists, rheumatologists, and oncologists, only to be given conflicting diagnoses and advice. Finally, some progress was made when "the diagnosis of a rare blood condition that a hematologist monitored but did not treat" finally occurred. But the hematologist got it all wrong, it turned out. Only after consulting another hematologist at Loma Linda University Cancer Center was the correct diagnosis of a slow-growing form of B cell lymphoma made. The patient told this new doctor "what the (original) hematologist had been saying for more than a year: (the patient) did not have cancer and that monitoring was the best course of action." The patient eventually got the proper treatment but the reporter was careful to note that "the agonizing nerve damage to his (the patient's) hands and feet continues to plague him . . . the damage is probably irreversible . . . because his cancer went untreated for so long."

This is the perfect example of why, in cancer and autoimmune disease, misdiagnosis and lack of proper therapy can be devastating. The story drives home my point about the importance of an insistent, inquisitive, and aggressive attitude on the patient's part. It appears that, at least in twenty-first-century American medicine, you'd better watch out for yourself when it comes to receiving proper medical care, especially for those conditions that don't easily lend themselves to diagnosis.

Our mini–medical school coursework has covered a lot of ground, but we are not done yet. In Chapter 5, I talked about the issue of suicide, an entity that remains stubbornly and frighteningly fixed on our top ten killer's list. Even in 2020, seemingly educated and insightful people fail to grasp that psychiatric disease, like any other, has at its core a chemical basis. In my first year of medical school in Boston in the fall of 1979, along with my courses in anatomy, physiology, biochemistry, and microanatomy (histology), the people who designed the curriculum saw fit to include an individual course on depression. In my many years dealing with psychiatric patients and issues, I look back on that first course with almost a sense of amusement—that's how little, comparatively, was known about the neurochemical basis of psychiatric disease.

Psyche was the Greek goddess whose domain was the human soul. The website Greekgoddesses.fandom.com describes her as

> the goddess of the soul, spirit, and compassion. She married Eros, son of Aphrodite . . . her official Greek name means "the soul" or "breath."

Why the term *psychiatry* came about I cannot say, because any goddess of the soul seems to me to be more attached to religious significance than disorders of the mind. The term is said to have arisen in the mid-nineteenth century to form *psych-* (soul) and *-iatreia* (healing). Nevertheless, psychiatrists are all too familiar to patients in Western and industrial societies, and diseases of the mind are found in populations the world over. With reference to depression, 12.7% of Americans over age 12 have used an antidepressant medication in the past month, according to writer Lea Winerman in the November 2017 online issue of APA.org. That number increases to 19.1% for people over 60 and represents a 64% increase in the number of patients using these medications between 1999 and 2014.

I am not a psychiatrist, psycho-pharmacologist, or therapist, but I can tell you that the neurochemical that is the basis of treating depression has changed dramatically since I was in medical school. Whereas the course I took in school focused on the neurotransmitters norepinephrine and dopamine, it was not until 1987 that Prozac was introduced, the first drug to primarily deal with the neurotransmitter serotonin. So knowing that a major depressive disorder, which affects about 14% of the population, and a major depressive episode (about 16.5%, which is often found in patients with bipolar disease) is a major contributor to suicide, mental health professionals have used their research skills to create medications that will beneficially effect the complex neurochemistry in the depressed patient's brain.

When I was in school, there were basically two main classes of antidepressants: monoamine oxidase inhibitors (MAO inhibitors) and tricyclic antidepressants (TCAs). They came with their own set of bothersome side effects. But with Prozac, the first commercially available SSRI (selective serotonin reuptake inhibitor), a new way of chemically dealing with depression was born. You may have heard of these latter generation brand examples, such as Luvox, Zoloft, Paxil, Celexa, and Lexapro. Indeed, there are still others. But neuropharmacology research continued unabated. Later research efforts led to other classes of antidepressants, whose mechanisms of action were different than the SSRIs. Bupropion (Wellbutrin) was one of them. Another class that came along was the SNRIs (serotonin-norepinephrine reuptake inhibitors), such as Cymbalta and Effexor. Still later came ketamine, a drug I discuss in detail elsewhere in this book.

I am not trying to offer an extensive and detailed description of the nature and treatment of MDD, a major contributor to suicide, but to reiterate that the pharmacologic basis of treating this disease has changed substantially. In general, although the newer medications appear to offer a less onerous side-effect profile than their MAO and TCA predecessors, that does not mean that present pharmacotherapy for depression is without its challenges. You probably know from personal experience that finding an antidepressant medication that works for you or someone you care about is often a trial-and-error affair. It is probably the rule rather than the exception that you have to go through a number of trials of medications to find one that helps the depression (and often the accompanying anxiety, what doctors like to call a "comorbidity") and has a tolerable side-effect profile. As one psychiatrist I know put it: "You have to break some eggs to make an omelette."

I would never agree with opinions like Tom Cruise's, who famously weighed in on antidepressants on *The Oprah Winfrey Show* in 2005:

> . . . it is not a cure and is actually lethal. These drugs are dangerous . . . when you talk about emotional chemical imbalances in people, there's no science behind that.

People have been helped and lives have been saved, without doubt, through the use of antidepressant medication. Period. But that is not to say that other modalities to treat depression and anxiety are not worth examining, and the American Psychiatric Association has weighed in on this. In their PTSD Guidelines for patients and families, they conclude:

- Cognitive behavioral therapy (CBT) and/or psychotherapy in combination may be more beneficial than either treatment by itself for depression.
- For anxiety CBT, antidepressants and anti-anxiety medications have all been shown to be helpful. Psychotherapy is more effective than medications, and adding medication does not significantly improve outcomes compared to psychotherapy alone.

And what about CBT, an area of psychological care that is receiving increased attention recently? It and the related dialectical behavioral therapy (DBT) share a basis for personality disorders and mental pathology that is described in terms of a biosocial theory. In essence, this theory examines the interface between human biology and environment and looks carefully at what was first described in borderline personality disorder as a problem of emotional regulation. But whereas DBT arose as a form of therapy that was a derivative of CBT, adding the practices of acceptance, distress-tolerance, and mindful awareness, CBT began by addressing cognitive distortions, encouraging coping strategies, and examining the interplay between thoughts, feeling, and behaviors. Both therapies have been shown to be of benefit in a number of psychiatric disorders, including depression, anxiety, substance abuse, borderline personality disorder, and others. Scientists have found that there is evidence that CBT alone can be as effective in treating mild to moderate depression, PTSD, and anxiety, and when used with medication, it can be most beneficial in treating major depressive disorder. So compelling is CBT in treating emotional disease that there are reports that brain chemistry and neural (nervous-system-related) pathways are actually positively altered with its use.

I have attempted here to examine the most frequently encountered diseases and conditions that affect us. I regret that I cannot cover more of the pathology that plagues us in a book of this scope and size. In the Afterword section of this work, I hope to summarize where we have been, where we are going, and what we can do, from a personal and public policy point of view, in order to head off what looks to be a coming disaster in American health and healthcare. Unfortunately, the ramifications of the recent and ongoing COVID-19 pandemic is just one indicator of how stressed our medical system is and how poorly our leadership—and we ourselves—have responded to this crisis.

CHAPTER 12

What Is the Worst and Best That's Happened in Medicine and Healthcare Since I Graduated Medical School

The year 2019 marked a personal milestone: I retired from clinical medicine after 35 years. If you were to count the years I spent as a child rounding in hospitals with my late father, I spent over five decades seeing sick people in hospitals and other clinical settings. In that time, so much has changed about the practice and process of medicine and medical care.

In this chapter, I will first speak of the not-so-positive, and then the more positive, trends I have observed. Although these observations merely reflect my own experience, solid tendencies appear to have arisen in parallel with the novel and ingenious therapies that have helped so many patients.

The Most Disturbing Trends in Medicine and Healthcare

- **Doctors don't know as much as you think.** There's a pervasive perception among nonmedical people that doctors know it all. After all, don't they train for years, speak a secret language, and deal with fancy equipment and life-altering pharmaceuticals? While all of that may be true, doctors still, in many ways, are not perfect. They make mistakes in diagnosis and treatment. Just look at the opioid crisis. Yes, a large part of that was due to pressure from the drugmakers, but doctors had to buy into that. Without doctors prescribing, the crisis could never have happened. Doctors have long been put on a pedestal, and that's not really a good thing. Doctors certainly do great things, but they are human.

- **Patients rely too much on medication.** I have a great friend. He has been so for 35 years. He is smart, sensitive, educated, and a consummate professional. And yet when he was diagnosed with coronary artery disease and told by his physician that, after his angioplasty and statin therapy he could "do what he wanted," he reverted right back to his terrible diet of refined sugars, refined starch, and saturated fat. His mentality was "as long as I take the medication, the doctor said I can do as I please!" This dangerous and backward attitude is all too present among patients. Instead of wisely changing his lifestyle for the better, he chose to rely on medications, with their potential for side effects, to clean up the mess left by his bad habits.

- **Doctors don't listen to their patients as much as they used to.** Doctors more than ever are under time constraints. Because of demographic changes, doctors need to see more patients in less time with greater efficiency. The art of medicine has become the corporate business of medicine. It was not so in my father's time in medicine, where he would actually talk with his patients, eye to eye, and attempt to understand the whole person. Today, the "clinician" is playing jazz on the keyboard as she listens to you, barely making eye contact. A lot is lost in that approach, but I have no sure-fire answers as to how to fix it. However, I do have some advice.

- **Patients are rapidly leading to their own demise.** I've beat this dead horse until I can no longer lift my arms, and I will preach it wherever and whenever I can: The obesity epidemic, fueled by a horrible diet and sedentary lifestyle, is the most dangerous threat to public health since smoking cigarettes became widespread. Perhaps even more so. In article after article, video after video, I have warned patients that obesity and its sister conditions are so very detrimental to health that its importance cannot be overestimated. Patients are truly digging their own graves with a knife and fork, adding high blood pressure, diabetes, joint disease, cardiovascular disease, and cancer to their list of obesity-related maladies on their diagnosis list. And it gets worse with each passing year. If I were a presidential candidate, I would beat the warning drums about this major American disaster, which costs us all over a trillion dollars a year and make attacking this scourge a top priority.

Despite all this, people continue to complain and moan about "their right to healthcare." However, no one I know discusses from whence this right derives. Even if we assume there *is* something close to a "right" to anything (fish have no "right" to fly, nor birds to live underwater, or for me to play tennis like Roger Federer), there must also be, naturally, personal responsibilities that go along with this.

As I've stressed, ad nauseum, medical science is chock-full of studies linking overweight conditions and obesity to myriad health problems: high blood pressure, diabetes, cardiovascular disease, autoimmune disease, cancer, and other bad things. The number of prescription medicines the average American takes is growing as well, reflecting the trend in increasing weight. Small wonder there's a correlation. Human physiology was not designed to withstand the highly caloric, sedentary lifestyle that is common today.

And yet, people cry out for relief of their self-induced maladies. Why is this? For starters, it is easy to lose sight of what constitutes good health and nutrition habits if one is constantly bombarded by a "foodie" tilted media. At no time in history have so many calories been so cheap. One can go to any number of fast food "restaurants" and get 3,000 calories for less than $3. As well, it takes effort to eat intelligently and exercise.

And this trend has had a recent impact. Writing in the April 20, 2020 edition of the *New York Times*, reporter Jane Brody presented the following horrifying facts, communicated by researcher Dr. Dariush Mozaffarian:

> Dr. Mozaffarian explained that poor metabolic health was the immunity-impairing factor underlying cardiovascular disease, Type 2 diabetes, and obesity-related cancers that left so many nutritionally compromised Americans especially vulnerable to the lethal coronavirus now all but paralyzing the country. "Only 12% of Americans are without high blood pressure, high cholesterol, diabetes, or pre-diabetes," he said in the interview. The statistics are horrifying, but unlike COVID, they happened gradually enough that people just shrugged their shoulders. However, beyond age, these are the biggest risk factors for illness and death from COVID-19.

This is a terrifying finding and confirms the major premise of my book. I applaud the reporter and Dr. Mozaffarian for bringing this wake-up call to light, but I harbor no delusions that the public will heed the warnings.

Let's be honest, most people, when left to their own preferences, would rather sit on the couch and each potato chips than eat and act as they know they should. The proof? Just look around you. Look at the covers of the magazines in the checkout aisle of the supermarket. They're all about dieting and losing weight. You can't watch TV for more than 10 minutes without seeing an ad for prescription medicines, diet plans, appetite suppressants, and junk food. Our society is saturated with both the cause *and* the supposed cures for this problem.

Some people might think that what I'm saying here is politically incorrect. As a physician who daily sees people wreck their health I say, "Get over it. Too bad." It's time to take off the gloves.

With the federal budget allocated to healthcare now topping a trillion dollars per year, it's time to be blunt. If you, the American patient, want to rid yourself and the nation of the health and financial suffering inherent in the present state of affairs, embrace the simple truths: Calories consumed must be fewer than calories expended. Ditch the refined sugar. Work out. Take responsibility.

According to the CDC, the combined cases of syphilis, gonorrhea, and chlamydia reached an all-time high in 2018. Consistent with that, I was surprised and concerned to receive a report around that time from the department of health in my home state (Maryland) on the national and statewide increase in the cases of syphilis reported in the past few years. This sexually transmitted disease, not often seen in recent decades, has made an unfortunate resurgence due to a number of factors that I will describe next. But first, let's talk about the disease itself.

The condition, in its primary, secondary, and tertiary forms, is caused by a corkscrew-shaped microorganism called a spirochete, an ugly little bacterium that goes by the Latin name *Treponema pallidum*. Like its nasty cousins gonorrhea and chlamydia, syphilis is an STD—a sexually transmitted disease. With sexual contact, particularly that where men have unprotected sex with other men, and where people exchange sex for drugs, the incidence nationwide increased a whopping 78% between 2012 and 2016. Sadly, the disease can be spread to newborns in the birthing process, where the incidence has increased 88% during this same time. This has been due to the alarming increase in the infection among young women. Clearly, we have a national problem.

What does one look for in this condition? The primary and secondary disease reveals:

- Painless genital or oral ulcers (called chancres)
- A rash on the palms or soles of the feet (macabrely known as the "Hollywood Measles" in the 1920s and 30s)
- Genital warts
- Patchy hair loss and overall body rash

The tertiary stage means central nervous system involvement (the stage Al Capone had when he died, as did Vladimir Lenin, Scott Joplin, and Howard Hughes), with difficulty walking, mental and behavioral changes, and other neuro/psychiatric manifestations.

There is a blood test for the disease, but up to 30% of patients can still have it and get back a negative blood test.

The good news is that injected penicillin is a great cure. The bad news is that many people have the disease and don't know it. So may all their sexual partners.

Why the increase in incidence? Other than the factors mentioned earlier, be aware that online dating and hookup sites are likely to blame. The population is letting its guard down, it seems, concerning safe-sex practices. So what should be done?

- Use common sense and discretion.
- Practice safe sex.
- Get tested if you have any signs or symptoms.
- Talk to your doctor.

Remember: Biology does not care if you are rich, famous, or educated. Your bloodstream is still a great swimming pool for spirochetes.

Emergency Room Wait Times and Overcrowding Are Getting Worse

One universal complaint among patients today is that the wait to be seen, or the time one stays in the emergency rooms of hospitals, is so long. This has been an issue for a while, but it appears to be getting worse. The questions are "Why?" and "What can be done about it?"

First, understand that emergency rooms (ERs), also called emergency departments (EDs) and emergency wards (EWs), are a microcosm of the healthcare system. Also know that 70% to 80% of hospitalized patients come in through the ER. *That is a huge number.* There are so many factors that are at play in delays related to this area of the hospital, it is hard to know where to begin.

The ER is the major gateway to the hospital. This gateway is being impacted by:

- An aging and more chronically ill population
- A shortage of nursing and ancillary staff
- A relative shortage of doctors

- A policy that forbids turning anyone away from the ER for care
- Triage—the system by which a member of the staff (usually the triage nurse), assesses the severity of a person's condition and allocates the speed and intensity of care accordingly
- Obamacare, which has given many more Americans access to the hospital
- The fact that people are using the ER as a main source of their primary care, either because they don't have a doctor or they cannot see one soon enough because of delays in getting appointments

These are all major factors as to why ERs are so overcrowded, under-staffed, and full of waits and delays.

Another factor is that hospital beds are in demand, and in order to admit a patient to the hospital, a bed must be made available. This does not always occur in a regularly smooth way, and delays are inevitable.

When one realizes that in a given community, one-quarter of the population in any given year will visit the ER as a patient, it is not difficult to see why access to timely ER visits is problematic. In high tourism areas, the number increases to one-third of the population.

Once in the system, other problems arise that are representative of the complexity and multifactorial reliability of the cogs in the hospital machinery. A patient who finally gets admitted may need lab tests (one source of potential delay), a CT or MRI scan (another source of delay), to be seen by a specialist (still another delay), intra-ER procedures to be performed (insertion of IVs, insertion of bladder catheters, nasogastric tubes, suturing of wounds, transfusion of blood, the list goes on), and finally, to wait for a bed to open up in the appropriate area of the hospital.

That means that many times the ER ends up being its own ward, a boarding area to handle all of the overflow that is an inherent result of the system.

And guess what? All this leads, as one might expect, to a high burnout rate among all the members of the ER staff. This burnout serves only to exacerbate the problem, and so the vicious cycle continues.

So what steps can you take to help yourself and others who truly need the ER? Consider the following:

- Avoid, if at all possible, using the ER as a primary care venue.
- Try as best you can to schedule doctor office visits well in advance. Also, choose doctors, if possible, whose schedules are more open, even if it means driving extra distances.
- Consider telemedicine options and email to get care, if your doctor or insurance company offers that.
- Be very specific when talking to the triage nurse about the severity of your symptoms. This is crucial in proper and more rapid allocation of care.
- Always carry your essential information—insurance card, brief medical history, a list of medications, and allergies and sensitivities you have, so there are no delays when you go to the ER.
- Have a patient advocate—a spouse, family member or friend—who can assist you, if possible.
- Take better care of yourself so you won't get sick. I mean this—this is not a joke. Lose weight, stop smoking, meditate, exercise, and keep your friends close. This is the best strategy of all, and it's all free.
- Prednisone continues to be overprescribed. Prednisone is a steroid medication used to treat a variety of ailments and is

instrumental in dealing with serious autoimmune, respiratory, endocrine, and other disorders. However, because its effects are so powerful and rapid-acting, it has been the source of medically induced injury and patient abuse for decades.

Used to rapidly "quiet down" inflammatory processes, prednisone carries a host of side effects that can be quite serious. These include exacerbation of high blood pressure, diabetes, gastrointestinal problems, anxiety and other psychiatric disorders, insomnia, and loss of bone density. Also, higher doses of prednisone may alter your physical appearance, leading to fat collection in your face and the back of your neck, as well as the waist and trunk, and cause a loss of muscle mass, too. When used in the short term, prednisone's benefits may outweigh any negative side effects. However, when used long term, for months or more, the unwanted effects are often worse than the disease it is designed to mitigate. I'd advise you to always ask your doctor if the benefits of this powerful drug outweigh the risks. And do realize that if you are on prednisone for an extended period, you may have to be weaned down from the peak dose in order to avoid an adrenal crisis, where your adrenal glands cannot produce enough of your own corticosteroids to meet the demands your body makes.

To illustrate the dangers of prednisone abuse, I will relate the story of a friend who had had some of the medication left over from a prior ailment. He decided, without telling his doctor, to start using the leftover pills as anti-inflammatory medication to treat his lower back pain. The result? His diabetes and blood pressure got so out of control that he ended up with a serious infection, developed septic shock, and eventually succumbed to the complications of his actions. This is a clear example of how prednisone must always be prescribed carefully and thoughtfully, and that any serious side effects of the medication must be addressed.

- People still suffer from postdural puncture headaches (PDPHs) at a higher-than-necessary rate, especially after diagnostic spinal taps from neurologists and after C-section anesthesia.

In the modern surgical and anesthesia era, millions of patients worldwide have been safely anesthetized with either spinal or epidural anesthesia. The theory behind these forms of anesthesia is simple: The anesthesiologist or other practitioner gains access to the adjacent nerves and anatomical region near the sac that encompasses the spinal cord and injects local anesthesia there to render the body area below that level insensitive to pain. In the case of *epidural* anesthesia, the numbing medication is injected superficial (more toward the surface of the body) to where the spinal fluid is, in a space called the *epidural space*. In the case of *spinal* anesthesia, the medication is delivered deeper (more anatomically beneath the surface of the body), to where the spinal fluid resides, in a space called the *subarachnoid space*.

But whichever type of anesthesia the provider chooses—spinal or epidural—there is the potential to create a complication known as a postdural puncture headache (PDPH). A PDPH is a bothersome and at times debilitating occurrence. This complication seems to be particularly more common among new mothers who delivered by C-section or had an epidural for a conventional delivery. It is also common in patients who have had a diagnostic spinal tap from a neurologist. It can occur in one of two ways. The first way is from an epidural anesthetic whose needle went too deeply and punctured the space that contains the spinal fluid—in the parlance of anesthesiologists, a "wet tap." The second way PDPHs can develop are from spinal anesthesia itself. Certain people may just be prone to developing them, even when flawless technique is employed.

A PDPH is characteristic in that it disappears when the patient is lying down, only to reappear upon sitting up or standing. It can be accompanied by ringing in the ears, light sensitivity, and nausea, and the headache can be most pronounced in the back of the head. It is a truly miserable experience and many patients have come to me for a certain treatment for relief that I discuss next.

Certain risk factors exist for the development of PDPH from spinal anesthesia. Younger patients tend to get it more frequently and severely than older ones. Also, the type of needle used by the anesthesia provider can have a great impact on the development of PDPH. The larger the bore of the needle, the greater the chance of PDPH. That's why you should always ask any provider, particularly if you are in your 20s or 30s, to use a needle of greater than 22 gauge—that is, request a needle of 25 or 27 gauge. The higher the number, the thinner the needle and the less chance of getting a PDPH. You'd think you would not have to ask, but do so! Sometimes doctors need reminding, if you can believe that.

The type of needle is crucial as well. Ask for a *Sprotte* or *Whitacre* needle if those are available. They have a bevel design on the tip that creates a puncture whose shape is much less conducive to developing PDPHs. You see, it is the hole in the punctured membrane that can cause a continuous leak of spinal fluid and lead to the brain literally sagging in the skull, causing the headache and symptoms I've described. That hole usually closes on its own but in some cases stays open from a "wet tap" epidural or spinal anesthetic, leading to a PDPH and its attendant miseries.

If a PDPH develops and is resistant to bed rest, fluids, caffeine (a traditional treatment option), and pain medicine, an *epidural blood patch* might be necessary. That is accomplished by doing an epidural and then "patching" the dural puncture hole with the patient's own blood, which is drawn in advance from the arm. The blood creates a clot that fills and closes the hole, thereby sealing the leak. After blood patching, patients are so relieved and happy to be rid of their headache that these are some of the most grateful patients one can imagine. As I recall, all of the patients I've treated with a blood patch have been women.

So remember: if you are going to receive spinal anesthesia (which by the way, in appropriately chosen patients, is a great anesthetic), go for the thinnest needle, a Sprotte or Whitacre tip, and seek out the most skilled provider you can find. And do realize that even in the best of hands, epidural anesthesia can result in a "wet tap," perhaps necessitating the blood patch "cure."

The COVID-19 Pandemic

The COVID-19 pandemic has caused unprecedented physical, mental, emotional, and economic suffering, and has painfully revealed the cracks and flaws in the American healthcare system. Any quotes here of the number of patients testing positive for the novel coronavirus, the number of related deaths, the economic impact in jobs lost, the debt accrued in government assistance and stimulus would be pointless because the figures change with each passing day. There are so many disturbing things about the pandemic it is hard to know where to begin.

The 2020 COVID-19 pandemic, by any measures, has been disastrous for our country and the world. I will not debate the nuances of whether the pandemic has been underplayed or overplayed in the press, the merits or lack thereof of the efforts employed by agencies and officials across all levels of government, if wearing masks outside in public while keeping a distance of at least 6 feet is too cautious or not cautious enough or any other points you might want to argue. I will leave that for the scientists, sociologists, activists, politicians, reporters, and pundits to hash out later.

What I will say is this: The United States, like a boxer with his hands down, was unprepared for this and got smacked. Hard. You might have thought that the implications of Hurricane Maria from September of 2017 would have offered an ample warning, but it did not. Referring to that natural disaster's effect on the nation's supply of intravenous fluid, the *Guardian* noted in a January 10, 2018 article by Julia Carrie Wong that Baxter International had 100% of its mini-bag IV solutions made in factories in Puerto Rico. That's right: 100%. Said pharmacy director Dr. Rita Jew of the University of California San Francisco Mission Bay Hospital:

> It really doesn't speak well to our healthcare system at
> this point.... A lot of people are referring to this like
> it's almost a third-world country, and there's some truth
> to that. These are basic supplies that we have taken for
> granted. It's kind of like we're rationing water in the U.S.

I remember that, at the time, these shortages were making their presence known in my own clinical work, and I had the same thoughts. "Third-world country" was the phrase I kept repeating to myself. I wondered at the time how ironic it was that a nation that never seemed to have a shortage of tobacco, soft drinks, razor blades, and bourbon suddenly could not supply a product as crucial but as simple as sterile salt or sugar water. I was dumbfounded.

And it was not just IV solutions that were in short supply. Injectable local anesthetics, like lidocaine, bupivacaine, and carbocaine, which have been in clinical use in the United States for more than 50 years and are staples of the anesthesia, surgery, and general medical communities, suddenly couldn't be found either. It was as if I was practicing on some distant third-world planet, where the basic tools of my profession were nowhere to be found.

In light of these revelations, it is not difficult to understand why our country's response to the pandemic has been so chaotic, ineffective, and if the statistics are accurate, deadly.

I say "if the statistics are accurate," because there is reporting out there that claims that COVID-19 deaths are not accounted for accurately. People say all kinds of things: That hospitals and healthcare institutions receive more government subsidies or other funds if a death is declared to be a result of a novel coronavirus infection, that if one member of a household is infected, it is assumed that all members of the same household are infected, and so on. I am no conspiracy theorist and these claims might appear to some to be preposterous. But it is important to seek valid, objective information that supports or refutes these ideas in order to uncover the truth.

I have no idea if any of these statements are true or not, and neither do you. The truth, unfortunately, appears to be in short supply these days. But still, there are clinical scenarios that are hard to deny. The virus is very contagious. It is quite dangerous in the elderly, the chronically sick, and the immune-compromised. It can cause very serious and apparently long-lasting disease in what were thought to be nonvulnerable patient populations. It does very strange things to the human body. In some patients, most notably the younger ones, the entity we now call *cytokine storm* can wreak havoc. The National Cancer Institute defines this as

> a severe immune reaction in which the body releases too many cytokines in the blood too quickly. Cytokines play an important role in normal immune responses, but having a large amount of them released all at once can be harmful.... Signs and symptoms include high fever, inflammation ... and severe fatigue and nausea. Sometimes a cytokine storm may be life-threatening and lead to multiple organ failure.

And that's not all this unpredictable pathogen can do. There are reports of strokes, due to coagulation (clotting) disorders found in the blood of patients in all age groups, most startlingly in younger patients. Scientists have reported the presence of megakaryocytes, the precursor cells to the blood-clotting element in the blood called platelets, in a range of tissues in patients who have experienced strokes. These tissues, mostly the heart, lungs, liver, kidneys, and brain, do not normally harbor that specific type of cell and it surprised investigators to see them there. To some pathologists and other doctors who study it, these reports are reminiscent of the dengue fever infections of the 1960s, a tropical disease transmitted by virus-carrying mosquitoes. Simply put, it is believed that the present virus is somehow augmenting the effect of the platelets, causing enhanced coagulation and thereby an increased risk of stroke. In reality, the true pathophysiology is much more complicated than that, but suffice it to say that the coronavirus does some very strange things with respect to your body's clotting mechanism.

The full story of the pandemic will not be told for years, and debate will rage on over a number of topics, perhaps most prominently related to the handling of our response to it. But what is indisputable is that we were unprepared, lacking in coordination and at the mercy, once again in human history, of nature. Humankind has suffered worse and will in the future, but to many it sure does not look like that from where we stand. By the middle of July 2020, trends began to emerge that confirmed what many experts had feared. The gradual (and not so gradual) easing of restrictions, particularly in the southern and western states, had caused a resurgence in infection and an uptick in the death rates. HealthTap reported in its July 11, 2020 Saturday Digest that Arizona, Florida, and Texas were seeing what it called "dramatic" increases in case rates and the beginnings of rising death rates. They observed that 89% of Arizona

ICU beds, 85% of Florida ICU beds, and roughly 86% of Texas ICU beds were in use at the time of that report.

The same day that the HealthTap report was published, a story from the *Washington Post* by Lena H. Sun lent credence to one major premise of this book: We do not merely have a healthcare crisis in the United States, but a health crisis. In particular, this was reflected in the fact that minority patients were suffering higher rates of serious complications and death from the coronavirus than their nonminority cohorts, confirming the CDC's statement that "some minorities experience a disproportionate burden of preventable disease, death, and disability compared with non-minorities." Ms. Sun confirmed that sentiment by observing the CDC's own analysis of 52,000 confirmed deaths between February and April of 2020, which found the following:

- There was a higher death rate among certain racial and ethnic groups.
- Among whites, the median death age was 81, among Hispanics it was 71, and for all non-white non-Hispanics it was 72.
- 35% of Hispanics who died were younger than 65, 29.5% of non-white, non-Hispanics who died were under 65, and 13.2% of deaths in whites occurred under the age of 65.
- The percentages of deaths among Hispanic and non-white, non-Hispanic people exceeded their representation in the U.S. population.
- Deaths in patients over 65 were skewed as well, where 41% were white, 21% were Hispanic, and 32% were non-white non-Hispanic.

The reporter also stated that a prior CDC report concluded that "people with . . . conditions such as heart disease and diabetes were hospitalized six times as often as otherwise healthy individuals infected with the coronavirus during the first four months of the pandemic and they died 12 times as often" from the virus.

Sleep Apnea

The incidence of obstructive sleep apnea in our country continues to rise. According to a 2014 report from the American Academy of Sleep Medicine (AASM), 25 million adults suffer from OSA (obstructive sleep apnea), a disorder they link to an increased risk of high blood pressure, heart disease, type 2 diabetes, stroke, and depression. They note that the *American Journal of Epidemiology* published studies revealing that the disease has "increased substantially over the last two decades, most likely due to the obesity epidemic."

The then president of the organization, AASM, was dire in his assessment:

> Obstructive sleep apnea is destroying the health of millions
> of Americans, and the problem has only gotten worse over
> the last two decades. The effective treatment of sleep apnea
> is one of the keys to success as our nation attempts to
> reduce health care spending and improve chronic disease
> management.

A 2015 review article on the subject in the *Journal of Thoracic Disease* was equally bleak, where authors Karl A. Franklin and Eva Lindberg concluded:

> OSA is highly prevalent. . . . Only a part of subjects with
> OSA . . . have symptoms in the form of daytime sleepiness.
> The prevalence of OSA and OSA syndrome has increased
> in studies . . . over time. Cardiovascular disease, especially

stroke is related to OSA and subjects under 70 run an increased risk of early death if they suffer from OSA.

That is why it is so important to get evaluated by a physician if you suspect you or a loved one is suffering from it. Risk factors include the following:

- Obesity, although not everyone with OSA is obese or even overweight
- Hypertension
- Smoking
- A chronically stuffed nose
- Having a family member with OSA

Mayoclinic.org says to be watchful for the following:

- Excessive daytime sleepiness
- Loud snoring
- Episodes of observed cessation of breathing
- Awakening with gasping or choking
- Difficulty concentrating
- High blood pressure
- Sweating at night

There are effective treatments for OSA, and there are things you can do to reduce your risk. Losing weight is one of them. CPAP (continuous positive airway pressure) masks can reduce your risk of complications and can save your life. But you have to take the first step and see a doctor if you suspect you may have OSA.

Electronic Health Records (EHRs)

The advent of the electronic health record (EHR) or electronic medical record (EMR) has streamlined and simplified communication about your health and medical history, including lab data, radiology, and other imaging reports, as well as vaccinations, medication lists, prior surgeries, medical conditions, and other data vital to treating you in the best possible way. These records are being mandated by certain government agencies and third-party payors; I'd be surprised if you didn't have one by now.

According to the website gminsights.com, "Increasing healthcare expenditure will stimulate the global EHR industry," with the market size in 2018 of $25.5 billion expected to rise to $38 billion by 2025. Other than increased healthcare expenditures as reasons for growth, they cite "growing funding and initiatives for implementation of EHR, enhanced patient care, and implementation of national strategies" as drivers for this growth.

But whatever the forces driving the increase in the use of EHRs, you should realize one important thing: EHRs, like any medical records, are only as valuable as the accuracy of the information in them. That is why it's crucial that you periodically review the contents of your EHR with your doctor in order to verify the accuracy of its content. In particular, you should attend to your major diagnoses, medication lists, and list of surgeries and procedures, as well as any legal documents (advanced directives, powers of attorney, etc.) that may be part of your records.

You should also find out if doctors and other medical professionals outside of your primary network will be able to access or interface with your existing EHR. Oftentimes, this is not the case, and it is better to find out as soon as possible in order to arrange for records to be shared most effectively with caretakers who are not privy to your EHR.

My Favorite Advances in Medicine and Healthcare

This last section will cover some of my favorite medical advances of the last 50 years.

- **Americans are smoking far fewer cigarettes** when compared to decades ago. According to the CDC, a mere 14% of Americans smoked in 2017, an impressive 67% reduction in smoking from its high point in the 1960s. That is huge. Reflected in this is the vast decrease in cardiovascular disease deaths during that time. Death from stroke, a major risk of smoking, has decreased 75% over that same time frame. (Now, if only we could get a handle on the obesity epidemic, then we really will have accomplished a lot.)

- **Life expectancy for Americans increased** 6.6 years between 1970 and 2005. Since 2005, the numbers have gotten even better (until recently among certain demographics). Again, less smoking has a lot to do with this, but better diagnosis and treatment of cardiovascular disease has contributed to it as well. However, don't think of this as final. Obesity and overweight rates of over 70% still threaten to undo or mitigate some of those advances.

- **New therapies, like gene therapy and stem cell therapy**, show promise for diseases as diverse as sickle cell anemia, Parkinson's, ALS, cancer, autoimmune disease, heart disease, type 1 diabetes, and others. Gene therapy involves introducing genetic material into a target cell to replace or block a protein that causes a disease state. Stem cell therapy, controversial in its own right (see my prior criticism on unregulated and sham forms of this technology), has shown promise when properly developed and employed by legitimate university-based or NIH-affiliated research centers. It is a complicated topic to discuss scientifically, but one could easily learn the basics behind this multifaceted therapy by reading various resources on the web.

- **Genetic testing has saved and improved lives.** Tests exist now that were not available decades ago. Bipolar disease, certain cancers, Parkinson's, celiac disease, Tay-Sachs disease, cystic fibrosis and many neurologic diseases, as well as others, are amenable to genetic testing. Early diagnosis and treatment were key to helping so many people suffering from these diseases and conditions before this technology came along.

- **Telemedicine** is something that really was only a dream decades ago. Now, people who don't have easy access to care, and even patients in busy urban areas who can't get an appointment with their doctors, are still able to get the attention they need in order to address many medical issues that require follow-up. This trend appears only to be growing. The recent COVID-19 pandemic has showcased the superb advantages of telemedicine. There are still kinks in the system, but overall this has been a boon to patients everywhere.

- **Medical care delivery by physician's assistants and nurse practitioners** is a growing trend, and this has helped greatly in the delivery of healthcare for many straightforward medical problems. Despite the boons here, I am convinced these professionals are best utilized when physicians carefully oversee their activities. A September 10, 2019 *Medscape* article on the topic of diagnostic error by Marcia Frellick reported that "Poll results indicated that NPs and PAs . . . reported slightly higher rates of daily diagnostic uncertainty than did physicians." But NPs and PAs, like physicians, are only as diagnostically skilled as their training, knowledge base, and index of suspicion (see Chapter 7) will allow.

- **The internet** can be a boon for research into medical problems and where to get care for the discerning consumer. But beware of the "Dr. Google" syndrome, and don't try to diagnose yourself. Seek professional help before you draw conclusions.

- **The CAT scan, MRI, and PET scan.** Whatever would we do without them? Before these more advanced methods of anatomical imaging, doctors had to rely on now seemingly primitive and more invasive methods to see the body's internal structures. Believe it or not, in order to visualize the brain and other physical elements of the central nervous system, doctors used to perform pneumoencephalography, a technique whereby air, helium, or oxygen was injected into the space where spinal fluid had been removed, and the patient was rotated any number of ways, assuming uncomfortable positions and often enduring postprocedure headaches and vomiting (see my description of postdural puncture headaches earlier in this chapter). To visualize joint spaces, like the knee or shoulder joint, doctors would perform arthrograms, where a suitable contrast material was injected into a joint space and then analyzed using a standard X-ray imaging technique. I had one myself for a knee injury in the 1970s, and let me tell you, it was not a pleasant experience.

  Nowadays, doctors use these advanced techniques to visualize in exquisite detail any number of internal structures and organs. With PET scanning (positron emission tomography) doctors are able to actually see the chemical activity your body is performing in real time, particularly in reference to cancer, heart function, and brain dysfunction. PET scanning is often used in conjunction with CAT scanning and MRI; the technologies can have a synergistic effect when used to diagnose certain conditions and best formulate a proper treatment plan. It is not an exaggeration to say that these imaging breakthroughs have saved untold lives and improved the chances for recovery in millions of patients worldwide.

- **The rise of transcranial magnetic stimulation (TMS)** for depression, anxiety, and other mental health disorders. Simply put, this FDA-approved therapy employs the use of targeted magnetic fields to create brain-specific electrical currents. These currents in turn result in the alteration of neurotransmitter release across the synapses, which is a fancy way of saying that "feel-good" chemicals are increased in the brain and central nervous system. The technique is considered to be noninvasive and is generally well-tolerated, although infrequent side effects can be fainting and seizures. There is potential application here for other disorders, including migraines, autism, bipolar disease, PTSD, Parkinson's disease, ALS, schizophrenia, and as an adjunct to help in quitting smoking.

- **3-D organ printing is becoming a thing.** Research is ongoing into the possible printing, using alginate (a gummy substance derived from the cell walls of brown algae) or fibrin polymers as a skeletal base for various organs such as the heart, liver, kidney, urinary bladder, or esophagus in transplantation medicine. There are still many kinks in the process but research in this area is showing clinical promise.

- **Cardiac surgery has changed for the better and has become less invasive** in many cases. Consider this celebrity example. As 75-year-old Mick Jagger, the frontman for the Rolling Stones might tell you, no one is immune to the ravages of time (or lifestyle). When it was announced recently that he was to undergo open heart surgery, many people not in the medical profession showed they didn't know what that actually meant.

For instance, does open heart surgery always mean that the doctors "open the heart"? Or can it mean opening the chest to get to the heart? Well, it depends on the procedure, the doctor, the health of the patient, and the technology available. Basically, open heart surgery, where cardiopulmonary bypass, better known merely as "bypass," is or isn't used, usually refers to two major types of heart surgery: valvular or artery. Sometimes, doctors perform both.

With our Western lifestyles and diets, coronary arteries, the vessels that supply the blood and therefore oxygen to the heart muscle to keep it vital and healthy, can become blocked with plaque, a gritty, fatty material derived from cholesterol and clotting elements. Doctors, for decades, have honed their skills in building new highways of blood flow around these blocked areas by using bypass grafts, which are usually vessels taken from the leg or chest. In this way, new pathways are formed to revitalize ailing heart muscle. This can be done, depending on the specifics, either the "old" way by splitting the sternum, or breastbone, or by going through the spaces between the ribs, considered "minimally invasive" techniques.

The heart has four valves—aortic, mitral, tricuspid, and pulmonic—and these can suffer from varying states of disease due to different causes. These causes can be infectious, genetic, traumatic, or be related to a host of medical conditions. When replacing or repairing valves, cardiac surgeons use prosthetic valves, derived from naturally occurring or synthetic products. Valve surgery can be done through the sternum or the spaces between the ribs, depending on the factors listed earlier, and be performed, if necessary, concomitantly with coronary artery surgery.

Lesser publicized surgeries in the heart involve the closure of passageways between the chambers that, through anatomic variation or disease, cause a disruption of heart function.

When talking about open heart surgery, be sure to know the what, how, where, and why before you jump to any conclusions. Also realize that cardiopulmonary bypass (where the heart is stopped, ventilation is stopped, and the blood is oxygenated by a machine outside of the body) is not always used. Check with your doctor about this if and when the topic comes up. But keep in mind that more noninvasive techniques to handle your cardiac issue may be available.

- **The Interstate Medical Licensure Compact (IMLC)** has made it easier for doctors to get licensed in other states. Since January 2019, 25 states, Washington, DC, and Guam reached an agreement with the Federation of State Medical Boards to enable doctors to practice in the states and areas that are part of the agreement. The states that are part of this compact are Alabama, Arizona, Colorado, Idaho, Illinois, Iowa, Kansas, Maine, Maryland, Michigan, Montana, Nebraska, Nevada, New Hampshire, Pennsylvania, South Dakota, Tennessee, Utah, Vermont, Washington, West Virginia, Wisconsin, and Wyoming.

  Unless you have practiced medicine, you do not understand the complexities and challenges faced when attempting to gain licensure in certain states. I will not name the worst offenders, but there are horror stories out there of qualified and talented physicians waiting years to obtain licenses due to clerical ineptitude, laziness, and just plain vindictiveness on the part of state medical boards. And if that weren't enough, the information requested is often so nitpicky in nature and onerous to obtain as to border on the absurd. I am not talking here about copies of medical school diplomas; internship, residency, and fellowship certificates;

board certifications; and continuing medical education doc-
umentation, which in and of themselves should be sufficient.
No, I am referring to the following: copies of medical school
transcripts, standardized medical examination scores, letters
of recommendation, criminal background checks, proof of
privileges and employment in *every* hospital, clinic, office
setting, and medical institution you ever practiced in or at,
and any number of other redundant minutiae.

Now, with the IMLC in place, these gathered documents have been centralized and the agreement allows for
licensure in other states other than the original certifying
state. This means, obviously, that whenever a qualified doctor
wants to practice in another state, she or he does not have to
regather all the necessary documents that are requested and
hope that the people responsible for sending and collating
the requested materials follow through and the clerical
workers do not screw up the process.

The clear winners here are patients. We have covered in
this book the doctor shortage in this country and it is only
going to get worse. The existence of the IMLC will allow
for easier licensure in states with underserved areas, and
that can only be a good thing. In fact, the U.S. Congress
should compel the remaining states to join the compact so
that more easily obtainable licensure is available to doctors
nationwide. Patients need this now and in the future.

- **The curing of hepatitis C** has been nothing short of a
medical miracle and is a shining example of the adage that if
you throw enough money and brainpower at a problem, you
are likely to achieve great things. Hepatitis C, like hepatitis A and B, is a viral disease that affects liver function. The
baby boom generation has been particularly hard hit with
chronic hepatitis C infections, many of which were related

to intravenous drug abuse and sexual transmission. It is estimated that the rate of acute hepatitis C illness that is self-limiting is in the minority and that 75% to 85% of people infected with hepatitis C will go on to have chronic disease. And of those people with chronic disease, a significant portion of them will develop serious sequelae (complications), such as scarring (cirrhosis), liver failure, and even liver cancer.

In cases of gradual fibrosis and scarring of the liver, the website liverfoundation.org says that after years of quiescence, patients may experience the following:

- Fatigue
- Weight loss
- Nausea
- Abdominal pain
- Itching
- Jaundice, or yellow discoloration of the skin and eyes

People at risk, the website says, are:

- Injectors or snorters of unclean needles and straws
- People who have gotten tattoos with unsterile equipment
- Healthcare workers who have been exposed to the virus
- Blood transfusion or organ transplant recipients before July 1992
- Clotting factor recipients before 1987
- Hemodialysis patients
- Children of infected mothers
- People who had unprotected sex with multiple partners
- People who had sexually transmitted diseases
- Patients with HIV

Unlike hepatitis A and B, there is no vaccine to protect against hepatitis C, but there are drug regimens that offer the chance of a cure. A cure is defined in this sense as a sustained virologic response, where no virus is detected in your bloodstream three months after the completion of the treatment. The antiviral therapies used to cure hepatitis C are not without the potential for risk and side effects and must be carefully coordinated—depending on the specific nature of your disease and your general health—by your doctor and the team taking care of you.

You should always be mindful of the costs involved in the therapy and be in close contact with your insurer or health plan before and during treatment. As reported by Maggie Fox from a May 6, 2018 NBC News article, the costs can be staggering. The article states that for the 3.5 million people infected (and half are not even aware of the infection), over 90% can expect to be cured, but at great expense. Matt Salo, of the National Association of Medicaid Directors had this to say: "There are probably a million people who have hepatitis C in the Medicaid world. . . . When it costs $64,000 to cure hepatitis C, that's a great deal. Multiply that by a million people? That's what makes people freak out."

- **HIV infection is no longer a death sentence**, at least in areas where patients are privy to appropriate care. As with the curing of hepatitis C, money and scientific sweat are behind the remarkable story of treating what was once the most feared new disease to come along in years. I can remember being a third-year medical student doing my internal medicine rotation in the wards of University Hospital in Boston when the buzz started about patients presenting with a rare form of pneumonia. Fast forward to today, and in retrospect the little we knew about what was first described as HTLV-III, now properly referred to as HIV, is almost embarrassing.

I will not cover the long history of the discovery and treatment efforts of the virus that causes AIDS other than to say, in passing, that I have a personal connection to the codiscoverer of HIV, Dr. Robert Gallo, a family friend. I can remember taking my little cassette recorder to his office at the NIH in the early 1990s in the hopes of writing a freelance story, based on that interview, on the status of the disease at that time. No publisher ever took me up on the effort, but I was and am grateful to Dr. Gallo for his friendship and enormous contributions to the health and betterment of so many people.

Although great strides have been made, HIV infection is still quite serious for people unable to get full access to care. Writing in ourworldindata.org, writers Max Rosner and Hannah Ritchie reveal that:

- Almost a million people worldwide still die from the infection.
- In some nations, it is responsible for one-quarter of all deaths.
- Death rates are high among younger adults.

But the brighter news is that:

- In the last 10 years, global deaths from HIV infection have been cut in half.
- Antiretroviral therapy prevents 1.2 million deaths per year.
- Life expectancy in Sub-Saharan Africa is now back to pre-epidemic levels.

Despite all the good news about HIV, we cannot let our guard down. About 1.2 million Americans still harbor the virus, and 1 out of 7 of them do not even know it. The CDC reports that in 2018, 76% of HIV patients received some care, 58% were kept in care, and 65% had the virus suppressed or it was undetectable.

Even so, these treatment figures are impressive and reflect the great efforts that have been put forth to stop a virus that had, decades ago, an entire nation and world terrified.

Afterword

What are we to make of a situation where the wealthiest and most powerful nation in the world, a country that spends the most per capita on healthcare ($10,209 per person in 2017—$2,000 more than the second-place country, Switzerland), has such poor health outcomes? What does it reveal about both our health and our healthcare system when a pandemic like that of COVID-19 wreaked such havoc here and has brought our nation to its knees? Will we ever learn the lessons we need to in order to reign in our out of control healthcare spending, improve the quality of our lives in our later years, and help prevent the chronic diseases that are even now affecting our younger people?

The answers to these questions lie between the covers of this book. Our health habits are abysmal. Period. Our diets and physical activity regimens are very much out of tune with natural human biology, which through evolution fine-tuned itself to foster a balance between the amount and type of calories we consumed with our physical efforts in obtaining those calories. Today, we are seeing the ravages of not hewing to the habits of our hunter–gatherer ancestors. Yes, I know we live in different times. I am fully aware that we cannot and never will go back to a way of life that has been extinct for thousands of years.

Technology and medicines have lengthened our lives and, under current social constructs, improved them by measures that are difficult to fully comprehend. But at what cost? I can tell you that the current trends are unsustainable—we will never be able to afford the ever-increasing costs of longevity and the chronic diseases that accompany it—unless some medical miracle comes along. As I have insisted throughout this book, only changes in attitudes and behaviors about who we are as biologically distinct animals in a complex world will mitigate the damage we have already inflicted upon ourselves.

The COVID-19 pandemic is a case in point. The issues related to that pandemic are so complex and so controversial that I will not even attempt to address a handful of them. I will say this: No one, and I mean no one, alive today knows the truth behind the novel coronavirus, because the truth, at this time, is unknowable. No one knows, for example, how many people have died *as a direct result* of COVID-19. It may be far more or less than the statistics touted. No one knows the true infection rate in a given population, and no one knows for certain what measures have or have not helped to prevent the spread of the infection. Common sense tells us that social distancing, mask wearing (in certain instances, not all), and sanitary methods such as handwashing appear to have been beneficial in "flattening the curve." The areas of the country that opened up in June and July of 2020 appear to have suffered from that easing of restrictions. In hindsight, the images of revelers crammed on the beach in Coney Island, New York, and in public places in Florida, Texas, Arizona, and California are cringeworthy now. What were people thinking? That they were immune from a virus shown to be more contagious than the flu and with a greater tendency toward unpredictably dangerous behavior?

But let us not lose sight of the lessons learned so far. COVID-19 was and is so deadly, if the mortality statistics are accurate, primarily because Americans are so chronically sick. Data from the June 24 edition of the *Economist* concurred:

> In hard-hit rich countries, about 60% of all deaths from the
> disease are among people 80 and older. America . . . is an

exception. Data released on June 16th by the CDC show that the country's death toll skews significantly younger. There, people in their 80s account for less than half of all COVID-19 deaths; people in their 40s, 50s, and 60s account for a significantly larger share of those who die.

And then the article offers conjecture as to why this is so. When I read it, I could only nod my head in understanding:

Why is America such an outlier? . . . Americans may be less healthy than their European peers, e.g., because they tend to be more obese.

What have I been saying all along? That obesity is the "mother of all diseases." That obesity places you at risk for hypertension, diabetes, acid reflux, cancer, degenerative joint disease, heart disease, and a host of other maladies. Because it is common knowledge that those individuals with chronic illnesses fare far worse when infected by COVID-19 than their healthier counterparts, a primary aspect to the answers we seek are staring us straight in the face.

Surely, it has to be more complex than that. There must be other answers, known and not known, as to why one person versus another would die from COVID-19. I am not saying obesity is the *only* factor in explaining the higher death rate among Americans. But sometimes the simplest answers are the compelling ones. It is something to consider carefully.

Scientists are now trying to formulate treatments and vaccines to help defeat the novel coronavirus. Here in my own backyard, the federal government just threw $1.6 billion at the Gaithersburg, Maryland, company Novavax, to develop a working vaccine and provide, by the start of 2021, one billion doses to the American public. Operation Warp Speed, the name of the federal project tasked with developing a vaccine for COVID-19, involved the spending of almost $4 billion in efforts to get America vaccinated. Alex Azar II, the U.S. Secretary of Health and Human Services said of this specific effort: "Adding Novavax's candidate to operation Warp Speed's diverse portfolio of vaccines increases the odds that we will have a safe, effective vaccine as soon as the end of this year."

There were reports as of July 2020 from the *New York Times* that as much as $10 billion would be appropriated by the U.S. Congress toward developing a vaccine against COVID-19. And while it can only be perceived—except to the anti-vaxxers among us—that a safe and effective vaccine is a good thing, it is once again a reminder of the frail nature of American health.

Here is another instance where our poor health habits are costing us, to the tune of 10 billion taxpayer dollars. I am not going to blame anyone or anything for the COVID-19 pandemic. I will, however, categorically state that the pandemic has been made worse by the poor general health of our population. You are free to draw your own conclusions.

The pandemic has taught us other bitter lessons as well. In the June 19, 2020 edition of the *Washington Post*, reporter Laurie McGinley wrote that "pandemic-related delays in diagnosis, treatment could be felt for years"with regard to cancer. Norman Sharpless, the director of the National Cancer Institute, noted that because of the pandemic, anywhere from 75% to 90% fewer mammograms and colonoscopies were performed, which is estimated to result in 10,000 excess cancer deaths from breast and colorectal cancer. He warned that "cancers missed now will come to light eventually, but at a later stage ('upstaging') and with worse prognoses."

And cancer care is not the only area of medical intervention that has worsened under the pandemic. The July 9 edition of the *Washington Post* noted a wave of opioid overdose patients flooding the healthcare system. Reporters William Wan and Heather Long said "Nationwide, federal and local officials are reporting alarming spikes in overdoses—a hidden epidemic within the coronavirus pandemic." But collateral effects were felt even earlier. In a May 7, 2020 article in Kaiser Health News written by Will Stone and Elly Yu, the authors noted that empty ERs worried doctors who felt potential stroke and heart attack victims were avoiding emergency care due to the pandemic. The authors reported that:

> The fallout from such fear (of COVID-19 infection) has concerned U.S. doctors . . . while they have tracked a worrying trend. As the . . . pandemic took hold, the number of patients showing up at hospitals with serious cardiovascular emergencies such as strokes and heart attacks shrank dramatically. . . . Across the U.S., doctors call the drop-off staggering, unlike anything they've seen. And they worry . . . people who have delayed care . . . will be sicker and [their] injuries will be exacerbated by the time they finally arrive.

Across the board, whether it be delayed dental care, cancer screening, diagnosis and treatment of acute cardiovascular emergencies, or other disruptions, patients are suffering and dying due to the ramifications and stresses imposed by the pandemic. It will be a long time indeed before we fully understand the full impact of what has befallen us.

So where do we go from here? The answers are clear. We have choices to make, and I am not optimistic. If we learn anything by the example set by the pandemic and the implications to our already inefficient and overstretched healthcare system it is this: You cannot expect the federal government, an HMO, a health insurer, or a healthcare provider to guarantee your health. It is one thing to pay for a health plan, earn a Medicare or veteran's entitlement, or shell out for a concierge doctor and expect decent basic health coverage.

It is quite another to expect that you will not pay the price, that *we* will not all pay the price, for the destructive habits we continue to embrace. But I harbor no delusions. I know what human nature is. I have seen it in almost four decades of dealing with patients. Many people who are much smarter and more influential than I have said similar things. Former FDA commissioner David Kessler wrote about the obesity problem in his 320-page 2009 book *The End of Overeating: Taking Control of the American Appetite*. Since that book was published, things have only gotten worse.

That does not mean I cannot try.

No, what it will take to effect true positive change is personal responsibility. You cannot expect things to improve if you yourself do not act. This is not a liberal versus conservative issue, a Democrat versus Republican issue, a racial or economic issue—it is a *personal choice* issue. That is not to say that there do not exist disparities in access to and quality of medical care across the spectrum of American life—many people, especially the poor, the uneducated, and minority groups are the first to suffer these privations. But no demographic of people, rich or poor, of any hue or religion, helps themselves by abusing their bodies.

If you learn nothing else from this book please try to incorporate these crucial messages: Keep your weight in the normal range, with a BMI of between 20 and 25. Limit your intake of processed food and saturated fats. Vary your diet, especially with foods of deep and rich natural colors. Try and keep your relationships close and meaningful. Do not smoke. Drink alcohol moderately and laugh a lot. Run if you can. If you can't do that, bike or swim. If you can't do that, walk. Lift some weights, twice or three times a week. Meditate. Consider, with your doctor, if you can get off of some of your medications. Consider supplements. Keep your friends close.

Good luck.

Index

About the Author

David Sherer, M.D., is an American physician, author, and blogger. His popular blog "What Your Doctor Isn't Telling You" appears monthly in Bottom Line Inc., a Connecticut-based publisher of books, web articles, and newsletters that provides advice from experts covering a range of health, business, personal, and other topics. HealthTap, a medical technology company based in Mountain View, California, has named Dr. Sherer for their leading anesthesiologist award twice.

Dr. Sherer retired from his clinical anesthesiology practice in the suburbs of Washington, DC, and now focuses on patient education, writing, and patient advocacy through his blogs, interviews, podcasts, and videos. Having appeared in all forms of media, he is a tireless advocate for patients and believes that personal responsibility, and not government intervention, is the key to improving the general health and well-being of all Americans.

More Titles From Humanix Books You May Be Interested In:

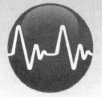

Simple **Heart Test**

Powered by Newsmaxhealth.com

FACT:

▶ Nearly half of those who die from heart attacks each year never showed prior symptoms of heart disease.

▶ If you suffer cardiac arrest outside of a hospital, you have just a 7% chance of survival.

Don't be caught off guard. Know your risk now.

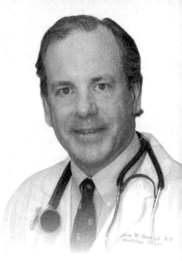

TAKE THE TEST NOW ...

Renowned cardiologist **Dr. Chauncey Crandall** has partnered with **Newsmaxhealth.com** to create a simple, easy-to-complete, online test that will help you understand your heart attack risk factors. Dr. Crandall is the author of the #1 best-seller *The Simple Heart Cure: The 90-Day Program to Stop and Reverse Heart Disease.*

Take Dr. Crandall's Simple Heart Test — it takes just 2 minutes or less to complete — it could save your life!

Discover your risk now.

- **Where you score on our unique heart disease risk scale**
- Which of your lifestyle habits really protect your heart
- **The true role your height and weight play in heart attack risk**
- Little-known conditions that impact heart health
- **Plus much more!**

SimpleHeartTest.com/Doctor